*Diabetes isn't a death sentence,
it's a wake-up call to live a healthier life.*
Kirt Tyson

# The RAWTRUTH

## THE RECIPE FOR REVERSING DIABETES

Ronnette,

Health is earned through sacrifice & knowledge.

Be Full of Life

## Kirt Tyson, N.M.D

The Raw Truth: The Recipe for Reversing Diabetes

Copyright © 2012 by Kirt Tyson, N.M.D.

All rights reserved. No part of this book may be reproduced in any form whatsoever, by photography or xerography or by any other means, by broadcast or transmissions, by translation into any kind of language, not by recording electronically or otherwise, without permission in writing from the author, except by a reviewer, who may quote brief passages in critical articles or reviews.

ISBN# 978-0-9855788-0-0

# Dedication

To anyone who has a desire to live and be healthy
by eating foods that give you life while preserving the lives
of other animals.

# Acknowledgements

I would like to thank the many people who have contributed to this book and the recipes. Special thanks to the chefs and raw food apprentices of Raw Life Café who helped me create and prepare the recipes in this book. These people include Kevin, Ben, Asia, Gretchen, Devin, Patrick, Afivi, and Danielle.

Special thanks to Kevin Covington for all the work he provided in gathering resources, taking pictures of the foods, and helping me to maintain balance while writing this book.

Without the support of my family and friends, this book would not be possible. A very special thank you to my dad, William Tyson, who encourages and supports me in every aspect of my life. Thank you Ahmed Allen, Audrey Oliver, Brian Henry, Carolyn Smith, Chyrus Founteno, Clarence Bryant, Clement Lee, Damien Patterson, Dorothy Hill, Florine Dirton Murray, Helen Tyson, Jerome Debro, Jerome Tyson, Keith Lyons, Kevin Darling, Liz Kim, Mark Burke, Mark Perlmutter, Roberta Parker, Ronald Malone, Tamaira Bailey, Terry Berry, Trina Savage Gardner, Ursula Fowlkes, and Wayne Christian.

Thank you to my very dear friend Marvin Williams for designing the cover. Thank you to the Mullins Creative team for editing and formatting the book. Thank you to Greyson Esprit for the additional pictures provided for this book.

Thank you to the many supporters of my film *Simply Raw: Reversing Diabetes in 30 Days*.

If there is anyone I forgot, please know that it was my memory and not my heart.

Kirt Tyson, N.M.D							www.livingrawforlife.com

# Table of Contents

**Preface** ..................................................................................................ix

**Chapter 1:** The Beginning............................................................................1

**Chapter 2:** Diabetes in Me .........................................................................5

**Chapter 3:** Becoming a Diabetes Expert ................................................11

**Chapter 4:** Diabetes Complications and Prevention .............................28

**Chapter 5:** Blessings from God................................................................31

**Chapter 6:** Experience at The Tree of Life..............................................36

**Chapter 7:** Experience in Naturopathic Medical School ......................38

**Chapter 8:** Rediscovery of Raw Foods ...................................................42

**Chapter 9:** The True Medical Model .......................................................46

**Chapter 10:** Escaping the Health Care Model .......................................58

**Chapter 11:** Detoxification........................................................................65

**Chapter 12:** Supplements .........................................................................70

**Chapter 13:** Plan of Action for Exercise..................................................76

**Chapter 14:** Living Raw for Life ...............................................................91

**Chapter 15:** Pulling it All together.........................................................100

The Raw Truth: The Recipe for Reversing Diabetes

**Raw Food Recipes** ...................................................................... **103**

**Bibliography** ............................................................................... **187**

# Preface

The body is capable of healing on its own once the obstacle to a cure is removed. This is seen in so many ways. When we cut ourselves, the cut heals on its own as long as we do not continue to pick at it as it heals. As amazing as the body is at remaining in balance and restoring health, it is difficult to believe that it cannot heal type 1 and type 2 diabetes.

Being diagnosed with diabetes and being told that there is no cure immediately sets up a road block in your mind, which results in hopelessness and despair. From my personal experience of reversing diabetes, however, I learned that the body is able to heal itself. That knowledge, combined with my medical training, led me to write this book.

This book will help restore your hope and belief that you can reverse diabetes without relying on medications. You will learn that diabetes is a condition that is within your control and you can take back your health. This book will help you to apply these principles of health to your life and share your new knowledge with your family and friends. As you reverse your diabetes, you will gain more energy and a longer life that you will be able to share with the people you love.

Having diabetes does not mean that you have to suffer and die. Yet this condition affects many people and its related complications are severe and debilitating. I do not want you to go down that same road.

As a physician, my practice focuses on getting people healthy, and I am regularly helping people reverse their disease. You have to know that you can beat diabetes. This book reaffirms that you are responsible for your own health. I can show you what it takes to be healthy, but you have to take the steps that will allow your body to heal.

**The Raw Truth: The Recipe for Reversing Diabetes**

I feel that this book is a comprehensive guide to reversing diabetes. It will help you to see how your attitude, thoughts, and relationship with food led to diabetes. It will give you the information you need to help you retrain your thinking and break the cycle of disease. And it shows you the steps you can take to reverse your diabetes.

This book has been six years in the making. I wanted to make sure that the recipe for reversing diabetes actually works, and time and time again I have seen people discontinue their medication, have their blood sugar levels stabilize to a normal level, and gain health and life. Through my own personal experience, I was able to see how my actions could keep diabetes away or bring it back. In this book, I'll share this experience with you.

# CHAPTER 1

## The Beginning

In the beginning God created the heavens and the earth. Provided that God exists in time, some scholars believe that one day for God is equal to one thousand years for man. It is generally accepted that the earth is about 4.5 to 4.6 billion years old. Calculations based on the Bible give the date for the creation of Adam and Eve as between 4,000 and 6,000 BC. Using the one day to one thousand year ratio, this equates to Adam and Eve being created 1.46 to 2.19 billion years ago. They are usually said to have lived 929 to 930 years, which in God's time is about 339 million years old. Since they were intended to be eternal beings, this longevity is to be expected.

In the creation story, God creates man and woman and says to them, "See, I give you every seed-bearing plant that is upon the earth, and every tree that has seed-bearing fruit, they shall be yours for food. And to all the animals on land, to all the birds of the sky, and to everything that creeps on earth, in which there is the breath of life, [I give] all the green plants for food" (Genesis 1:29). So clearly, ever since Adam and Eve defied God's wish for them not to eat the apple from the tree of knowledge, we have defied his every intent when it comes to eating. The biggest blasphemy against God is cooking food.

Based on our ratio of one day in God's time to a thousand years in human time, it would have been roughly 944 million years from the birth of Adam to the birth of Noah. That's enough time to do a lot to displease God and defy his wishes, so God decided to cleanse the earth and release a flood. It was after the flood that God said, in Genesis 9:3, "Everything that lives and moves shall be yours for food." This signifies a shift from a vegetarian diet to an omnivorous diet. It was also a time in which the life expectancy of a man was only one-third the length of the life expectancy of previous generations.

**The Raw Truth: The Recipe for Reversing Diabetes**

Roughly another 730 million years passed between Noah and Jesus. The period of time from the creation of Adam and Eve to the birth of Jesus accounts for about 1.7 billion years of history. Over time, man became distant from God and as a result, our concept of time changed. We no longer associated our measurement of time with God's timeline, but based it on the cycles of the world.

Our concept of time is based on what is relevant to us. One modern example of this is the country of Samoa, which just recently switched its time zone in order to be in the same time zone as a neighboring country with which Samoa conducts much of its business. They effectively skipped December 30, 2011 and went directly from December 29, 2011 to December 31, 2011.

Similarly, because our connection with God had diminished, we were willing to accept that the world was only 9,000 years old. In order to restore our belief in him, God sent his son Jesus. When we look at history with this new perspective on time, we can calculate that Jesus existed around 400 million years ago.

## Fire's Use Throughout History

Fire has been a part of the earth's natural landscape for about 400 million years, and volcanoes and lightning have been sources of wildfires for eons. When and how hominids evolved to eventually acquire the use, then subsequently the control, and finally the production of fire is subject to much speculation. Various anthropologists have pointed out that wildfires caused by lightning strikes are quite common in eastern Africa, and have been long before our human ancestors evolved to become capable of using these natural fires. Clear evidence also exists that humans are the only species to have developed this skill. Considering that the use of fire required a high intellect and that no antecedent species existed for early humans, it is reasonable to conclude that learning how to use fire was a slow historical process.

Today, fire plays an almost elemental part of everyday human culture. From the home furnace that heats the air to the gas stove used for cooking, we take the many uses of fire for granted. Think back to when you were a child and you tried to create fire in the backyard using two sticks. I rubbed for a long time and was never successful at creating fire; my closest success was making a piece of paper start smoking using the sun and a magnifying glass.

For early humans, it had to be a tough task to create fire with the wind blowing or during other less than ideal weather conditions. Even without those hindrances, using sticks, as opposed to matches or a lighter, to create fire is a heck of a task. Combined with the everyday dangers and necessities of survival, it would have been a huge chore indeed.

## Using Fire for Cooking

I'm sure humans have been using fire for millions of years out of necessity. Fire was probably one of the earliest of human discoveries, and would have initially been observed in nature. Natural causes of fire include lightning, sparks from falling rocks, volcanic activity, and the spontaneous combustion of plant materials and other organic matter. It is inaccurate to believe that humans' use of fire coincided with the use of cooking. In the beginning, fire may have only served to provide protection from carnivores and temporary warmth for our ancestors.

Brian Ludwig of Rutgers University conducted one study that supports this theory. Ludwig studied forty thousand pieces of flint tool artifacts, ranging from 1 million to 2.5 million years old, from sites throughout Africa, and found some surprising results. When rocks have been exposed to heat, they develop telltale signs of heat exposure, in the form of observable "potlid fractures." After studying his tool artifacts, Ludwig discovered that they started to show these small fractures only after about 1.6 million years. It was not until that time that Homo erectus was using fire for hunting and possibly using cooking tools.

Because the first fire residues in caves date to around 400,000 to 350,000 years ago, scientists conclude that this is when the long-term use of caves as dwellings began. The fire residues found inside these caves probably resulted from the use of controlled fire for light, warmth and warding off predators. No matter when it first occurred, it is safe to assume that its first users were not modern humans. One can imagine that the first successful spark was met with an enormous sense of pride, wonder, and happiness.

Changes in climate may have caused the widespread practice of cooking foods. The first modern humans, Homo sapiens, appeared between 140,000 and 110,000 years ago, which was also around the beginning of the last ice age. This drastic change in climate may well have triggered the widespread use of fire for warmth and cooking. So far we have been able to date the use of hearths (a term used for any deliberately constructed fireplace) to as far back as 125,000 years. The earliest known hearth is located at the Klasies River Caves in South Africa.

The question of how human beings first began using fire to cook food remains unanswered. Perhaps a hunter left one of his kills outside and it was frozen the next day, so he decided to throw it on the fire to warm it back up. Eventually the use of fire evolved into a process in which everything we eat is cooked. Clearly the first use of fire for cooking had to have been an accident, because we know how destructive fire is. Fire destroys; it burns houses, cars, clothes, money, and people. If we valued food and the essence it carries, we would not place it in fire.

# CHAPTER 2

# Diabetes in Me

I was born in Baltimore, Maryland on October 17, 1981. During this year the USDA found that people in the age groups of 25-34 and 50-64, with an above average income and a college education, were more likely to purchase and eat organic foods. In my case, however, I grew up in the inner city of Baltimore to low-income parents, so our food was provided by the government. This nutritious subsidy consisted of government cheese, peanut butter, whole milk, and butter. There were few resources promoting the health benefits of breastfeeding, so my mother opted to nourish me with cow's milk.

My exposure to the Standard American Diet (SAD) began at the age of five months. My parents had to make the best of an unfortunate situation that confronted many parents in my community. Since they had a very limited food budget, I was fed whatever was available. Typical meals included fried chicken, string beans, mashed potatoes and gravy along with bread.

Over time finances deteriorated even further, and we had to resort to eating syrup sandwiches and sugar water. The syrup sandwich simply consisted of King's Syrup poured on top of a piece of white bread. Sugar water is a liter of water with a cup of sugar. These meals provided the basis for the kind of diet I later deemed essential for survival.

During my childhood my main source of food was the school lunch program. Throughout much of middle school I was consistently ill and frequently got sent home because of my nausea and vomiting. Practically every time I ate pizza or chocolate milk at school, my stomach would ache and I would spend the rest of the day at the edge of the toilet. I later learned that I could not eat the school's pizza, and once I stopped eating the pizza, all of the symptoms subsided.

## The Raw Truth: The Recipe for Reversing Diabetes

During my freshman year of high school, I had a health class that aimed to teach students the benefits of eating healthy. Unfortunately for me, my idea of eating healthy consisted of sugar, sugar, and more sugar. Throughout most of high school, I ate hot dogs on a bun with ketchup, mustard, and relish. In high school and continuing into college, I ate fast foods and highly processed foods, including five pounds of duplex cookies a week.

I would also eat a bowl of cereal practically three times per day. I am not referring to Fiber One or Cheerios; I was eating Fruity Pebbles, Captain Crunch, Frosted Flakes, Lucky Charms, and Froot Loops. I was eating upwards of four pounds of these cereals each week, which amounted to roughly 768 grams of sugar. Over the course of a year, that would add up to 88 pounds of sugar. That total was just from cereal and didn't include the sugar from sodas and the other junk food I ate. I did a lot of intense activities; the sugar helped me to maintain what I believed to be optimal performance, so I continued eating this way. Unfortunately, my eating habits would get worse before they would get better.

The way I thought about nutrition was formed in my youth, when I didn't have the best diet and grew up believing that all I needed to survive was sugar. This idea was perpetuated during college. I majored in biology, and the courses I enrolled in included physiology, cell biology, and biochemistry. During my course of study I constantly learned about the importance of glucose (sugar) in producing ATP (energy) that enables our bodies to carry out life's processes. All cells need glucose to survive, and the brain uses sugar almost exclusively. So I believed that as long as I was eating sugar I was giving my body what it needed.

During my first two years of college I became a fast food junkie. I was eating fast food every single day at least twice per day. The workers at Popeye's, Wendy's, Subway, and McDonald's knew me on a first name basis. I would supersize all my meals; who could resist an order of extra large fries? My favorite meal was a bacon cheeseburger combo with a half and half (half sweet tea and half lemonade). The best half and halfs are in Baltimore; they have so much sugar in them that they could put anyone in a diabetic coma. I stayed away from soda because everyone always talked about how bad soda was for the body.

The after-hours place to eat was none other than The Waffle House. There I would order a Super All Star Special, which consisted of a waffle, three eggs scrambled hard with cheese, hash browns, grits, raisin toast, and two sausage patties. This combo was drizzled in butter and syrup. This food was good for the soul, even though most of the time I would feel tired and want to take a nap afterwards. Over time this effect made me concerned about my diet, but people told me that this was normal and everyone suffers from it. "The itus" was the term people used to describe this laziness one experiences after eating a big meal. Everyone experienced these same symptoms and never considered them a sign that anything was wrong, which led me to disregard my basic instincts. Therefore, I continued to eat the Standard American Diet and believed that what I was feeling was good and normal.

While in school I worked as a runway model, print model, and actor. To be successful in the entertainment business, you have to maintain a healthy appearance. I worked out daily, not necessarily to be healthy but in order to maintain a healthy-looking physique. I would run four to six miles per day, coupled with swimming and weight lifting. At that time, I stood six feet tall, weighed 175 pounds, and had eight percent body fat. I felt good and looked healthy. One of the top modeling agencies in the world, Elite Models, signed me, and I modeled for Urban Outfitters, Ralph Lauren, Jack Victor, and a host of other designers. As time went on, when I looked in the mirror, I saw myself as looking healthy, but I didn't feel healthy.

As I begin reading more and learning more about the body and its biochemistry, I started to question my eating habits. I asked my friends, family, and professors if eating large amounts of sugar caused diabetes, and everyone said no, eating sugar does not cause diabetes. I wasn't entirely convinced, so I started making dietary changes anyway.

I made small dietary changes over a period of a couple of weeks. I reduced the amount of cookies, milk, cereal, and red meats I ate and replaced them with chicken, tuna, salmon, and salads. I started feeling better and wasn't as sleepy after meals. I figured that I must be on the right path and finally felt like I was eating a healthy diet.

During the summer of 2005, I had an opportunity to work on the film Step Up while it was being filmed in Baltimore. Working on a major film comes with the benefits of craft services. Instead of breaking for breakfast, lunch, and dinner, food was provided throughout the whole day. It consisted of cookies, crackers, chips, soda, water, juice, fruit, bagels, and a host of other foods. Spending ten to twelve hours on set, I spent most of my time snacking as we waited to film each scene.

As weeks went by I found myself getting weaker. After a few weeks of filming I had gone from a person full of energy to someone who could barely move. I found that I would get tired unless I ate, so I ate constantly. Eventually, every time I ate I had to take a three to four hour nap. On Monday, I had to urinate quite frequently during the day and woke up twice at night to urinate. On Tuesday, I became so lethargic that I could barely walk up the steps after a meal and I woke up four times during the night to urinate. On Wednesday, I noticed that my vision had changed, I could no longer see the signs on the highway without squinting, and I was urinating every hour. I made an appointment with my optometrist, and he simply said that my vision had gotten weaker and wrote a stronger prescription for glasses and contacts. Thursday was the biggest wake-up call. I was sitting in class, and one of the girls came over to me and said, "You are really skinny; you look emaciated!" I was horrified and could not understand why she would say such a thing.

After class, I went to the gym and got on the scale. Just the week before I had weighed 174 pounds, but at that moment I was down to 154 pounds. I had lost 20 pounds in one week. I had no clue what was going on. By Thursday night I started tracking my urine output. From my medical training and courses in physiology, I knew normal urine output for an adult is 30-40 milliliters (ml) per hour, which equates to about 720-960 ml per day. I was urinating about 600 ml per hour, which is roughly 20 ounces. I couldn't drink enough water to keep up with the amount of urine I was putting out.

On Friday, I was scheduled to film again and would be doing part of one of the dance scenes. I made it to the set of Step Up, but I didn't have the energy to move around and was in no condition to film. At this point I was going to the bathroom every thirty minutes and was afraid that my kidneys were failing. I decided I needed to do something to boost my energy. That day, November 18, 2005, was the first time I had a Red Bull; it nearly gave me wings. I felt good for about an hour, and then I crashed. I could not move. I called the on-set medic, told him my symptoms, and they released me for the day. Once I was in my vehicle, I pushed the OnStar button, called my insurance company, and got authorization to go to the emergency room. That day I felt like I wasn't going to make it and I was on death's doorstep.

At the emergency room, I told the nurses my symptoms and waited for about ten minutes before they called my name. I went to the intake room and they took blood and vitals. Before I had a chance to walk back to the waiting room, the nurses called my name and took me immediately to the back. I was told that my blood sugar levels were too high to read on the meter.

I was in diabetic ketoacidosis, a condition that occurs when a person with diabetes becomes dehydrated. As part of the body's stress response, hormones (unopposed by insulin due to the person's insulin deficiency) begin to break down muscle, fat, and liver cells into glucose (sugar) and fatty acids for use as fuel. These hormones include glucagon, growth hormone, and adrenaline. These fatty acids are converted to ketones by a process called oxidation. The body consumes its own muscle, fat, and liver cells for fuel.

In diabetic ketoacidosis, the body shifts from its normal fed metabolism (using carbohydrates for fuel) to a fasting state (using fat for fuel). Blood sugar levels increase because insulin is unavailable to transport the sugar into cells for future use. As blood sugar levels rise, the kidneys cannot retain the extra sugar, which is dumped into the urine, increasing urination and causing dehydration. Usually, as a person slips into diabetic ketoacidosis they lose about ten percent of their body's fluids. Because of the excessive urination, significant loss of potassium and other salts is also common. Diabetic ketoacidosis is a severe condition and can result in coma or death.

I was started on fluids and insulin to reverse the ketoacidosis. It took three days in the Intensive Care Unit to get my blood sugar levels under control. While lying in the ICU, I was told that I had diabetes and I needed insulin. I was instructed how to inject myself with insulin. The doctor told me that this was a serious disorder and I would have to be on insulin for the rest of my life. I was left devastated and confused.

I honestly believed I had been living a healthy lifestyle. I ate relatively healthy, I had started avoiding red meat and opted for chicken and fish instead, and I exercised almost daily. How could it be that I had diabetes? As I lay there in the hospital bed, I prayed to God. I said, "Lord, if you help me overcome this disease, I will help others to do the same."

# CHAPTER 3

# Becoming a Diabetes Expert

**Anatomy and Physiology of the Pancreas**

The pancreas houses two distinctly different types of tissue. Most of its mass is exocrine tissue and associated ducts, which produce an alkaline fluid loaded with digestive enzymes. These enzymes include proteases to break down protein, lipases to break down fats, carbohydrases to break down carbohydrates, and nucleases to break down nucleic acids. This fluid is delivered to the small intestine to facilitate digestion of food.

The pancreas also contains several hundred thousand clusters of endocrine cells, which produce the hormones insulin, glucagon, and a few others. Insulin and glucagon are critical for glucose homeostasis and regulate blood glucose concentration. From a medical perspective, insulin is especially important; a deficiency in insulin or deficits in insulin responsiveness lead to the disease diabetes mellitus.

The pancreas is an elongated organ nestled next to the first part of the small intestine. In humans, the pancreas develops as an outgrowth of the duodenum, a part of the small intestine. The cells of both the exocrine system (the acinar cells) and of the endocrine system (the islet cells) seem to originate from the ductal cells during development. During development, these endocrine cells emerge from the pancreatic ducts and form aggregates that eventually constitute what is known as Islets of Langerhans.

Humans have four types of islet cells: the insulin-producing beta cells; the alpha cells, which produce glucagon; the delta cells, which secrete somatostatin; and the PP cells, which produce pancreatic polypeptide. In the human pancreas, 65 to 90 percent of islet cells are beta cells, 15 to 20 percent are alpha cells, 3 to 10 percent are delta cells, and one percent are PP cells. The hormones released from each type of islet cell have a role in regulating hormones released from other islet cells. These cells within the pancreas that synthesize and secrete hormones make up what we call the endocrine pancreas. The gross anatomy of the pancreas and the structure of pancreatic exocrine tissue and ducts are discussed in the context of the digestive system.

Nature loves order, which is why the different cell types within an islet are not randomly distributed: beta cells occupy the central portion of the islet and are surrounded by a "rind" of alpha and delta cells. Aside from the insulin, glucagon and somatostatin, a number of other hormones have been identified as products of pancreatic islet cells.

The products of islet cells are important and require the islets to be richly vascularized, meaning that they are well connected to the circulatory system, allowing the secreted hormones ready access to the rest of the body. Even though islet cells constitute only 1-2% of the mass of the pancreas, they receive about 10-15% of the pancreatic blood flow. Additionally, they are innervated by parasympathetic and sympathetic neurons, and signals from the nervous system clearly modulate the secretion of insulin and glucagon.

A loss of beta islet cell function is a contributing factor in diabetes. Dr. Ralph DeFronzo has stated that by the time diabetes is diagnosed, the patient has lost over 80 percent of beta islet cell function. This demonstrates how resilient the body is and how it works to maintain balance even in a less than ideal situation. The good news is that a loss of function does not mean that the cells are dead. Restoring function will restore the beta cells' ability to produce insulin.

## Structure of Insulin and Biosynthesis
Insulin is a rather small protein composed of two chains held together by disulfide bonds. The amino acid sequence is highly consistent among vertebrates, so that insulin from one mammal is almost certainly biologically active in another. Even today, many diabetic patients are treated with insulin extracted from pig pancreas.

In significant amounts, insulin is only produced in beta cells in the pancreas. The insulin mRNA is translated as a single chain precursor called preproinsulin, and removal of its signal peptide during insertion into the endoplasmic reticulum generates proinsulin.

Proinsulin consists of three domains: an amino-terminal B chain, a carboxy-terminal A chain, and a connecting peptide in the middle known as the C. peptide. Within the endoplasmic reticulum, proinsulin is exposed to several specific endopeptidases, which remove the C. peptide, thereby generating the mature form of insulin. In the cell's Golgi, insulin and free C. peptide are packaged into secretory granules, which accumulate in the cytoplasm.

When the beta cell is stimulated in the right way, it secretes insulin by exocytosis, and this insulin diffuses into islet capillary blood. C. peptide is also secreted into the blood, but it has no known biological activity. For this reason, tests measure the levels of C. peptide in the blood in order to determine how much insulin the pancreas produces or to distinguish type 1 from type 2 diabetes. Type 1 diabetics typically have low quantities of C. peptide, while type 2 diabetics typically have high quantities of C. peptide.

## Control of Insulin Secretion

Insulin is secreted primarily in response to elevated blood concentrations of glucose, since its role is to help the glucose to enter into the cells. Sight and smell can trigger insulin secretion, which can begin even before you take your first bite. We do not entirely understand the mechanism behind insulin secretion, but there are certain features of this process that have been clearly and repeatedly demonstrated. This model includes the following:

**Step 1:** Glucose is transported into the beta cell by facilitated diffusion through a glucose transporter. Elevated concentrations of glucose in extracellular fluid (fluid outside of the cell) lead to elevated concentrations of glucose within the cell.

**Step 2:** Elevated concentrations of glucose inside of the beta cell lead to membrane depolarization. As a result, calcium from outside of the cell (extracellular) floods into the cell (intracellular). This increase in intracellular calcium is thought to be one of the primary triggers for the exocytosis of insulin-containing secretory granules. Scientists are not entirely sure why elevated glucose levels within the beta cell cause depolarization, but they seem to be caused by metabolism of glucose and other fuel molecules within the cell. It's possible that the cell senses the shift in the ATP to ADP ratio, which then affects what kind of molecules move through the cell membrane.

**Step 3**: Increased glucose levels within beta cells may also activate calcium-independent pathways that participate in insulin secretion.

**Step 4**: The cell prepares to stimulate insulin secretion. The normal fasting blood glucose concentration in humans and most mammals is 80 to 90 mg/dl, and is associated with very low levels of insulin secretion.

**Step 5**: When the person takes in enough glucose to maintain blood levels two to three times the fasting level for an hour, then insulin is secreted. Almost immediately after the insulin begins spreading throughout the body, plasma insulin levels increase dramatically. This initial increase is because the cells are secreting preformed insulin, which is soon significantly depleted. The secondary rise in insulin reflects the considerable amount of newly synthesized insulin that is released immediately. Elevated glucose not only simulates insulin secretion, but also transcription of the insulin gene and translation of its mRNA.

## Blood Sugar Regulation

Glucose is the primary source of energy for the body's cells, and blood lipids (in the form of fats and oils) are primarily a compact energy store. The blood sugar concentration or blood glucose level is the amount of glucose (sugar) present in the blood of a human or animal. The human body naturally regulates blood glucose levels as a part of metabolic homeostasis. Normally, in mammals, the body maintains the blood glucose level at a range of between about 3.6 and 5.8 millimoles/liter (mmol/l), or 64.8 and 104.4 milligrams/deciliter (mg/dl).[2] The bloodstream transports glucose from the intestines or liver to the body's cells. The cells then use insulin to absorb the glucose. The mean normal blood glucose level in humans is about 4 mM (4 mmol/l or 72 mg/dl);[2] however, this level fluctuates throughout the day.

Glucose levels are usually lowest in the morning, before the first meal of the day. This is called the fasting glucose level. For an hour or two after meals, glucose levels are elevated by a few millimoles or milligrams. A high blood sugar level is referred to as hyperglycemia; a low blood sugar level is referred to as hypoglycemia. Severe stress, such as trauma, stroke, myocardial infarction, surgery, or illness, can temporarily increase the blood sugar level. Intake of alcohol causes an initial surge in blood sugar, and later tends to cause levels to fall.

Blood sugar levels are regulated by negative feedback in order to keep the body in homeostasis. The levels of glucose in the blood are monitored by the cells in the pancreas's islets of Langerhans. If the blood glucose level falls to a dangerous point, the alpha cells of the pancreas release glucagon, a hormone that causes liver cells to convert glycogen into glucose to increase blood glucose levels. The glucose is released into the bloodstream, increasing blood sugar levels. When levels of blood sugar rise, whether as a result of glycogen conversion or from digestion of a meal, a different hormone is released from beta cells found in the islets of Langerhans in the pancreas.

This hormone, insulin, causes the liver to convert more glucose into glycogen. (This process is called glycogenesis.) Insulin forces about two-thirds of the body's cells (primarily muscle and fat tissue cells) to take up glucose from the blood through the GLUT4 transporter, thus decreasing blood sugar. Insulin also provides important signals to several other body systems and is the chief regulatory metabolic control in humans.

## What is Diabetes?

Diabetes mellitus is characterized by persistent hyperglycemia from any of several causes, and is the most prominent disease related to failure of blood sugar regulation. It is classified as a metabolism disorder. Metabolism refers to the way our bodies use digested food for energy and growth.

When we eat, our body breaks down our food into simpler forms such as amino acids and glucose. Most of what we eat is broken down into glucose, which makes its way into our bloodstream as the food is digested. Our cells use the glucose for energy and growth. However, glucose cannot enter our cells without insulin being present – insulin makes it possible for our cells to take in the glucose. After eating, the pancreas automatically releases an adequate quantity of insulin to move the glucose present in our blood into the cells, and in this way it lowers the blood sugar level.

In the case of a person with diabetes, there is too much glucose in the blood, resulting in hyperglycemia. This condition occurs because the body either does not produce enough insulin, produces no insulin, or has cells that do not respond properly to the insulin the pancreas produces. As a result, too much glucose builds up in the bloodstream and it eventually passes out of the body in urine. So, even though the blood has plenty of glucose, the glucose does not help the cells meet their essential energy and growth requirements.

## The Origin of the Term "Diabetes"
Diabetes comes from Greek, and it means "siphon." Aretus the Cappadocian, a Greek physician during the second century AD, named the condition diabainein. He described patients who were passing too much water (polyuria) – like a siphon. The medieval Latin word "diabetes" was incorporated into the English language.

In 1675 Thomas Willis added "mellitus" to the term, although the disease is still commonly referred to simply as diabetes. "Mel" in Latin means "honey;" the urine and blood of people with diabetes has excess glucose, and glucose is sweet like honey. Diabetes mellitus could literally mean "siphoning off sweet water." In ancient China, people observed that ants would be attracted to some people's urine because it was sweet. The term "Sweet Urine Disease" was coined. In the African American community, diabetes mellitus is referred to as sugar diabetes or simply "sugar."

## Types of Diabetes

There are four main types of diabetes. The most common are type 1 diabetes and type 2 diabetes. The other types are gestational diabetes, which sometimes occurs during pregnancy, and type 1.5 diabetes. All types of diabetes mellitus result in too much glucose in the blood.

There are many factors that lead to the development of diabetes. When you look at the general causes of diabetes, you will find that the symptoms are always somehow related to lifestyle, heredity, and environmental factors. High sugar consumption is one of them. In type 2 diabetes, there are specific contributing factors, such as ethnicity, age, obesity, a sedentary lifestyle, pregnancy, and poor diet. Many studies find that there are genetic risk factors for type 1 and type 2 diabetes; however, those genes, such as the LD1 gene, are activated by a high fat diet.

## Type 1

Type 1 diabetes is an autoimmune disease: the person's body has destroyed his/her own insulin-producing beta cells in the pancreas. People with type 1 diabetes are unable to produce insulin. Type 1 diabetes used to be called juvenile diabetes or childhood diabetes. Now we simply refer to it as type 1 diabetes.

Most people with type 1 diabetes develop the condition before the age of forty. Developing type 1 after that age is extremely rare. The majority of people who develop type 1 are of normal weight and are otherwise healthy during onset. Quite simply, a person with this type of diabetes has lost his/her insulin-producing beta cells. Several clinical trials have attempted to find ways of preventing or slowing down the progress of type 1, but so far there has been no proven success. Approximately 15 percent of all people with diabetes have type 1. Type 1 diabetes is fatal if blood sugar levels are constantly elevated and the person does not take action to lower glucose levels, such as regularly taking exogenous insulin.

Type 1 diabetes is an autoimmune disease, which means the person's immune system mistakenly destroys the beta islet cells of the pancreas.

The body sees the cells as foreign invaders and attacks and kills them. Other autoimmune diseases include multiple sclerosis, lupus, Crohn's disease, scleroderma, and rheumatoid arthritis. Some autoimmune diseases are triggered by diet and lifestyle. This may be the case with type 1 diabetes. Some of the factors that seem to be linked to this disease include genetics, autoantibodies, viruses, drinking cow's milk, and oxygen free radicals.

Genetics is probably a factor in the development of type 1 diabetes. About ten percent of the population has genes that would result in type 1 diabetes; however, only one percent of those people actually develop type 1 diabetes. If the disease were purely genetic, you would expect the person's mother or father would have had diabetes as well. It is true that a child of a parent with type 1 diabetes is more likely to develop the disease than someone without a family history, but type 1 diabetes is not an inherited disease.

Some researchers believe a viral infection can trigger type 1 diabetes in people genetically vulnerable to the disease. In this scenario, the virus creates a viral protein that resembles the insulin-producing beta cell protein. This resemblance tricks the immune system, which then attacks the beta cells of the pancreas as well as the virus. Enteric viruses, so called because they are associated with human feces and attack the intestines, causing vomiting or diarrhea, are under particular scrutiny as a potential cause of type 1 diabetes.

Other researchers believe the trigger is actually casein, a protein in cow's milk. In infants that are feed cow's milk, the proteins are not fully digested, and amino acid fragments are left in the intestine and potentially absorbed into the blood. The immune system recognizes the foreign protein and destroys it; however, the protein being destroyed resembles the protein that makes up the beta islet cells of the pancreas. The immune system is no longer able to distinguish pancreatic cells from the foreign proteins and begins to destroy the pancreatic cells, which would lead to type 1 diabetes.

## Type 1.5 Diabetes

Previously there were only two recognized forms of diabetes: adult onset diabetes and childhood diabetes. As a result of modern changes in our environment and diet, children are now developing type 2 diabetes, which once only existed in adults. Additionally, in recent years scientists have identified several other diabetes subtypes beyond types 1 and 2. There is gestational diabetes, which resembles type 2 diabetes, appears during pregnancy, and can be harmful to the fetus; this type of diabetes disappears in the mother after childbirth. The most common "new" type of diabetes is called latent autoimmune diabetes in adults (LADA).

The term "type 1.5 diabetes" applies to diabetes cases diagnosed in adults who do not immediately require insulin for treatment, are often not overweight, and have little or no resistance to insulin. When special lab tests are done, patients are found to have antibodies, especially Glutamic Acid Decarboxylase 65 (GAD65) antibodies, that attack their beta islet cells. In addition to being called LADA, this sort of diabetes is also sometimes called slow onset type 1.

The first course of treatment may be diet, exercise, and standard type 2 medications, which are typically oral hypoglycemic drugs. Since insulin resistance is minimal or non-existent, medications designed to reduce insulin resistance, such as Metformin and Avandia, are not effective. Other medications that stimulate the pancreas to produce insulin, slow digestion of carbohydrates, or reduce excess glucose production by the liver are often effective in controlling the blood sugar for a few years.

LADA can be classified as a more slowly progressing variation of type 1 diabetes, yet it is often misdiagnosed as type 2. According to some estimates, around 15 to 20 percent of people diagnosed with type 2 diabetes actually have type 1.5 diabetes. The type 2 diagnosis is usually made because patients are older and will initially respond to diabetes medications because they have adequate insulin production and they are not resistant to insulin. There is still currently a lot of uncertainty over how exactly to define LADA, how it develops, and how important it is for patients to know if they have it.

Knowing whether you have LADA or type 2 diabetes truly is important, however, since management of the two conditions differs. For instance, type 1 diabetes, no matter the age of onset, requires a finely tuned insulin regimen. People with type 2 diabetes, on the other hand, sometimes do not need insulin at all, or when they do, they may need injections just once per day.

Doctors stumbled upon the LADA phenomenon quite by accident back in the 1970s while testing a way of identifying proteins called autoantibodies in the blood of people with type 1. The presence of these proteins is evidence of an attack by one's own immune system. The new test was successful and confirmed for the first time that type 1 is an autoimmune disease in which the body's immune system kills off the beta cells in the pancreas.

As part of their study, the researchers also looked for the same autoantibodies in the general population and in people with type 2 diabetes. The proteins were virtually absent in the general population, but they showed up, to the scientists' surprise, in about ten percent of people diagnosed with type 2. This suggested that there was a subcategory of people who could now be diagnosed as having LADA instead, even though there was no obvious difference in their symptoms from those people with type 2. Several other studies have shown similar results, and these studies also often show that antibodies, especially those against glutamic acid decarboxylase or GAD, which are characteristic of type 1 diabetes, are present in people diagnosed with type 2 diabetes.

Type 1.5 is a fitting term for this kind of diabetes. Researchers have found that genetically, LADA has features of both type 1 and type 2, including both autoantibodies and a genetic component. LADA appears to fall somewhere between types 1 and 2 on the diabetes spectrum, though it is perhaps closer to type 1.

## Type 2
Type 2 is the most common form of diabetes. The majority of people with type 2 develop the condition because they are overweight. Type 2 used to appear much later in life but is now being seen in children.

People with type 2 diabetes do not produce enough insulin, have decreased insulin receptors, or their body is resistant to insulin.

The most common features of type 2 diabetes are insulin resistance and elevated insulin in the blood. In the case of insulin resistance, the body is producing insulin, but insulin sensitivity is reduced and the process does not function as well as it should. Glucose does not enter the body's cells properly, which leads to a buildup of glucose in the blood and makes cells starve because they are not getting enough glucose. As the disease progresses, the person's insulin production is still not enough to lower their blood sugar levels and they often end up requiring exogenous insulin.

As previously stated, insulin is a hormone made in the pancreas that allows glucose to enter the cells to be used as fuel or be stored as fat. Type 2 diabetes occurs when the pancreas doesn't make enough insulin or the cells of the body become resistant to insulin. It is not known for certain why some people develop type 2 diabetes and some do not; however, there are several factors, such as genetics, obesity, and physical inactivity, that can increase a person's risk of developing type 2 diabetes.

Type 2 diabetes also involves problems with insulin receptors. Practically all cells in the body contain special proteins called receptors, which allow molecules to enter into the cell. They work like a lock and a key, with insulin as the key that binds to the receptors (the locks) on the cell's surface. In a healthy cell, this process causes GLUT4 glucose transporter molecules to come to the cell's surface. As their name implies, these glucose transporter proteins ferry glucose inside the cell.

If the insulin cannot first fit into the insulin receptor, however, then this process can't take place properly. In some cases people with type 2 diabetes have faulty locks that do not allow the insulin to fit. There also may not be enough receptors on the cell for insulin to bind to. In rare cases, the insulin is formed improperly and doesn't fit into the receptor. In all of the above situations, glucose is unable to enter into the cell and it builds up in the blood.

## The Raw Truth: The Recipe for Reversing Diabetes

There is a strong genetic factor in type 2 diabetes, meaning that people with close relatives with type 2 diabetes have a much higher incidence of developing it themselves. For instance, if one parent has type 2 diabetes, each child has about a 15 to 25 percent chance of developing it, depending on when the parent was diagnosed. If both parents have type 2 diabetes, there is about a 1 in 2 chance that their child will develop type 2 diabetes. Even though there is a big genetic link to type 2 diabetes, it is important to understand that those genes are activated by a diet with high fat and high animal protein intake.

Excess body fat increases insulin resistance and increases the risk of developing type 2 diabetes. One reason for this is that fat cells contain fewer insulin receptors than muscle cells. In addition, fat cells release free fatty acids, which also interfere with glucose metabolism. This is a vicious cycle because the glucose that is not metabolized by the body for energy is stored as fat, making more fat cells.

Over 80 percent of people with type 2 diabetes are overweight or obese. In obese individuals, fat is typically concentrated around the abdominal organs. It is this fat around the organs and not the subcutaneous fat that causes the organs to not function properly and may result in the development of type 2 diabetes. The fat around the waist secretes a group of hormones called adipokines, and this hormone may also impair glucose tolerance.

Other factors that are believed to contribute to type 2 diabetes may include low birth weight, age older than 65, or chronic stress. High stress raises production of a hormone called cortisol, which elevates blood sugar levels and requires more insulin to regulate blood sugar. Typically, high stress does not substantially affect blood sugar levels in people with normal insulin receptors.

Smoking is another factor that seems to increase the chances of developing type 2 diabetes. People who smoke have a higher rate of developing type 2 diabetes than people who never smoked. When people quit smoking, their risk for developing type 2 diabetes is higher for the first three years, but after ten years of being smoke-free the risk returns to the same level as that of people who never smoked.

## Gestational Diabetes

Almost all women have some degree of impaired glucose intolerance as a result of hormonal changes that occur during pregnancy. This means that their blood sugar may be higher than normal, but not high enough to constitute diabetes. During the third trimester, these hormonal changes place pregnant women at risk for gestational diabetes.

During pregnancy, increased levels of certain hormones made in the placenta help shift nutrients from the mother to the developing fetus. Other hormones are produced by the placenta to help prevent the mother from developing low blood sugar. They work by stopping the action of insulin. Over the course of the pregnancy, these hormones lead to progressively impaired glucose intolerance (higher blood sugar levels). To try to decrease blood sugar levels by getting glucose into the cells where they can be used as energy, the body makes more insulin.

Usually, the mother's pancreas is able to produce enough insulin to overcome the effect of the pregnancy hormones on blood sugar levels. If, however, the pancreas cannot produce enough insulin to overcome the effect of the increased hormones during pregnancy, blood sugar levels will rise, resulting in gestational diabetes.

Since gestational diabetes affects the mother in late pregnancy, after the baby's body has been formed, gestational diabetes does not cause the kinds of birth defects sometimes seen in babies whose mothers had diabetes before pregnancy. However, untreated or poorly controlled gestational diabetes can still hurt the baby. In the case of gestational diabetes, the pancreas works overtime to produce insulin, but the insulin does not lower blood glucose levels. Although insulin does not cross the placenta, glucose and other nutrients do. So the extra blood glucose goes through the placenta, giving the baby high blood glucose levels. This causes the baby's pancreas to make extra insulin to get rid of the blood glucose. Since the baby is getting more energy than it needs to grow and develop, the extra energy is stored as fat.

This can lead to macrosomia, or a "fat" baby. Babies with macrosomia face health problems of their own, including damage to their shoulders during birth. Because of the extra insulin made by the baby's pancreas, newborns may have very low blood glucose levels at birth and are also at higher risk for breathing problems. Babies with excess insulin become children who are at risk for obesity and adults who are at risk for type 2 diabetes.

## Symptoms of Diabetes

All people with diabetes have one thing in common: they have too much sugar, or glucose, in their blood. People with very high blood glucose levels share many similar symptoms:

- Extreme thirst
- Frequent urination
- Blurred vision
- Fatigue without an apparent cause

People with type 2 diabetes may also experience leg pain that may indicate nerve damage or poor circulation. Many people with type 1 and some people with type 2 diabetes experience weight loss even though they have an increased appetite and are eating more.

Over one-third of all people with type 2 diabetes are unaware they even have the disease. The nature of the condition makes it possible to have mild symptoms or no sign of type 2 diabetes for years before it is detected. In contrast, few cases of type 1 diabetes go undetected for long because the symptoms are severe enough that the individual will end up going to a doctor for help.

## Diagnosing Diabetes

The gold standard for diagnosing diabetes is an elevated blood sugar level after an overnight fast (not eating anything after midnight). The following tests are used:

## FPG Test

A fasting plasma glucose (FPG) test measures blood glucose in a person who has not eaten anything for at least eight hours. Results and their meanings are shown in Table 1. A value above 126 mg/dl on at least two occasions typically means a person has diabetes. A value above 100 mg/dl but less than 126 mg/dl on at least two occasions typically means a person is prediabetic. This result is also referred to as impaired fasting glucose (IFG) and means that the patient is at greater risk of developing type 2 diabetes. People with normal glucose metabolism have fasting sugar levels that generally run between 70 and 100 mg/dl.

The FPG test is used to detect diabetes and pre-diabetes. It is the preferred test for diagnosing diabetes because of its convenience and low cost. However, it will miss some diabetes or pre-diabetes that can be found with the OGTT.

## Table 1. FPG Test

| Diagnosis | Plasma Glucose Result (mg/dl) |
|---|---|
| Normal | 99 or below |
| Pre-Diabetes (impaired fasting glucose) | 100-125 |
| Diabetes * | 126 or above |

* This is confirmed by repeating the test a second time on a different day.

## OGTT

Research has shown that the OGTT is more sensitive than the FPG test and therefore can better diagnose pre-diabetes, but it is less convenient to administer. The OGTT requires fasting for at least eight hours before the test. The oral glucose tolerance test is conducted by measuring blood glucose levels five times over a period of three hours. An initial blood sugar measurement is drawn and then the person is given a "glucola" bottle with a high amount of sugar in it (75 grams of glucose or 100 grams for pregnant women). The person then has their blood tested again thirty minutes, one hour, two hours, and three hours after drinking the high glucose drink.

In a person without diabetes, the glucose levels in the blood rise after drinking the glucose drink. However, they fall quickly back to normal because the body produces insulin in response to the glucose, and the insulin then lowers the blood glucose level. In a diabetic, glucose levels rise higher than normal after drinking the glucose drink and come down to normal levels much slower. This is because insulin is either not produced, or it is produced but the body's cells do not respond to it.

Results and their meanings are shown in Table 2. If the blood glucose level is between 140 and 199 mg/dL two hours after drinking the liquid, the person has a form of pre-diabetes called impaired glucose tolerance (IGT). Having IGT, like having IFG, means a person has an increased risk of developing type 2 diabetes but does not have it yet. A two-hour glucose level of 200 mg/dL or above, confirmed by repeating the test on another day, means a person has diabetes.

For the test to give reliable results, you must be in good health (not have any other illnesses, not even a cold). Also, you should be normally active (for example, not lying down or confined to a bed like a patient in a hospital), and you should not be taking any medicines that could affect your blood glucose. The morning of the test, you should not smoke or drink coffee. During the test, you need to lie or sit quietly.

## Table 2. OGTT

| Diagnosis | 2-Hour Plasma Glucose Result (mg/dl) |
|---|---|
| Normal | 139 and below |
| Pre-Diabetes (impaired fasting glucose) | 140-199 |
| Diabetes * | 200 and above |

* This is confirmed after repeating the test a second time on a different day.

An Oral Glucose Tolerance Test can diagnose gestational diabetes by using 100 grams of glucose in the liquid the patient drinks. Blood glucose levels are checked four times during the test. If blood glucose levels are above normal at least twice during the test, the woman has gestational diabetes. Table 3 shows the above-normal OGTT results for gestational diabetes.

### Table 3. Gestational Diabetes: Above-Normal Results for the OGTT*

| When | Plasma Glucose Result (mg/dl) |
|---|---|
| Fasting | 95 or higher |
| At 1 hour | 180 or higher |
| At 2 hours | 155 or higher |
| At 3 hours | 140 or higher |

*These numbers are for a test using a drink with 100 grams of glucose.

### Random Plasma Glucose Test

A random plasma glucose test, also called a casual plasma glucose test, measures blood glucose without regard to when the person being tested last ate. This test, along with an assessment of symptoms, is used to diagnose diabetes but not pre-diabetes. However, blood glucose measurements during the oral glucose tolerance test can vary somewhat. For this reason, if the test shows that you have mildly elevated blood glucose levels, the doctor may run the test again to make sure the diagnosis is correct. A random, or casual, blood glucose level of 200 mg/dl or higher, plus the presence of symptoms, can mean a person has diabetes.

# CHAPTER 4

# Diabetes Complications and Prevention

In the weeks following my discharge from the hospital, I had a rude awakening. I didn't take my diabetes too seriously and actually started to care less about my health. I was bitter that I developed diabetes even after enacting changes in my eating habits and exercising.

My diet actually got worse. I ate whatever I felt like. I started eating red meat, cookies, milk, cheeses, and everything in between. I felt hopeless and did not believe that there was anything that I could do. So what was the point in trying? My doctor told me that no matter what I did I would have to take insulin for the rest of my life. I was taking 1000mg of Glucophage and 30 units of insulin daily and my blood sugar levels averaged 400 mg/dl (22mmol/l). I found myself spiraling out of control.

About three weeks after my diagnosis I received a phone call from my friend, who told me that his cousin had just died at the age of 22 from complications of diabetes. This man had been diagnosed with diabetes at the age of 10. He did not take insulin regularly, suffered from kidney failure, and required dialysis. He eventually died because his high blood sugar levels led to ketoacidosis that resulted in him becoming comatose and ultimately dying. It was a huge wake-up call for me. At that moment that I realized how serious and detrimental this disease is. He lost his life because he was not managing his diabetes and that was exactly what I was doing. I was, in essence, giving up my desire to live.

**Complications**
Diabetes causes more deaths every year than breast cancer and AIDS

combined. Two out of three people with diabetes die from heart disease or stroke.

While insulin allows a person with type 1 diabetes to stay alive, it does not cure the disease, nor does it prevent the development of serious complications, which can be many and varied. High blood sugar levels eventually damage blood vessels, nerves, and organ systems in the body. Among the potential complications of type 1 diabetes are:

## Cardiovascular Disease

Cardiovascular disease describes a range of blood vessel system diseases that includes both stroke and heart attack. It is the major cause of death in people with diabetes. The two most common types of cardiovascular disease are coronary heart disease, caused by fatty deposits in the arteries that feed the heart, and hypertension, or high blood pressure. Research shows that people with diabetes are more likely to have high cholesterol and hypertension, both of which cause damage to the cells lining the artery walls. Researchers think high blood glucose contributes to both of these conditions.

## Hypoglycemia

Hypoglycemia, low blood sugar, is a dangerous condition for people with diabetes. It can be triggered by not eating often enough, eating too little food, too much physical activity without eating, or too much insulin. People with diabetes can usually tell when their blood sugar is low. But the more episodes of hypoglycemia you have, the harder it gets for your body to detect the next episode. In severe forms, hypoglycemia can lead to unconsciousness or even death. For patients with type 1 diabetes, fear of hypoglycemia is a major obstacle to maintaining tight blood glucose control.

## Diabetic Kidney Disease

Diabetic kidney disease is one of the most common and most devastating complications of diabetes. It is a slow deterioration of the kidneys and kidney function that, in severe cases, can eventually result in kidney failure, also known as end-stage renal disease or ESRD. About one-third of people with type 1 diabetes develop diabetic kidney disease.

## Neuropathy

Neuropathy, or nerve damage, affects more than 60 percent of people with type 1 diabetes. The impact of nerve damage can range from slight inconvenience to major disability and even death. Diabetic neuropathy leads to loss of feeling and sometimes pain and weakness in the feet, legs, hands, and arms, and is the most common cause of non-accidental amputations in the United States.

In one type of neuropathy, known as autonomic neuropathy, high glucose levels injure the autonomic nervous system, which controls bodily functions such as breathing, circulation, urination, sexual function, temperature regulation, and digestion. Autonomic neuropathy may result in various types of digestive problems, diarrhea, erectile dysfunction, a rapid heartbeat, and low blood pressure.

## Retinopathy

Diabetic retinopathy is the most common and serious eye-related complication of diabetes. It is a progressive disease that destroys small blood vessels in the retina, eventually causing vision problems. In its most advanced form (known as "proliferative retinopathy") it can cause blindness. Nearly all people with type 1 diabetes show some symptoms of diabetic retinopathy, usually after about twenty years of living with diabetes; approximately 20 to 30 percent of them develop the advanced form.

# CHAPTER 5

# Blessings from God

I had been dealing with my diagnosis of diabetes for a little over a month, and my health was suffering. My blood sugar levels were constantly above 500mg/dl and I was having terrible headaches. I really felt hopeless and had no clue what I was supposed to do and how to do it. I was following the American Diabetes Association food guide for diabetics, but it still did not help me to regulate my blood sugar levels. Again, I asked God for help because I did not want to die so young.

My prayers were answered. I was searching the craigslist classifieds website looking for acting and modeling opportunities around Baltimore when I came across an advertisement seeking type 2 diabetics to participate in a documentary on reversing diabetes using raw foods. My eyes immediately lit up and I looked at the screen, knowing that my prayers were being answered. I took no time in responding to the craigslist post.

On January 5, 2006, I received an email in response.

> Kirt,
>
> Thanks for writing about this project. I'm a casting director on *Raw for 30 Days*, a film documentary shooting later this month in AZ.
>
> We are sending 5 people with type 2 diabetes to The Tree of Life center in AZ for 30 days, starting this month on the 21st. Participants will eat the raw food diet. It's an amazing opportunity (that normally costs $10,000 for one month) that few will be chosen to do. If you're available between then and Feb. 23, please fill out the attached application TODAY.

> If you would please fill it out on your computer and email us back, that would be terrific. We don't have time now to wait for mailed copies as we are making our decisions this weekend.
>
> Thanks for your interest. We hope to hear from you!

I was so excited to have heard back from them. I responded to the email that same day. When God sends you a blessing, you don't take your time to decide if you want to accept it or not. This was my application for the documentary:

1. Describe briefly your eating habits:

   **Breakfast**
   *Egg with cheese, toast, diet jelly, turkey bacon, piece of fruit*

   **Lunch**
   *Salad, small piece of baked chicken*

   **Afternoon**

   **Dinner**
   *Chicken breast, salad, greens, bread, salmon*

   **Snacks**
   *Turkey sandwich*

   **Favorites***

2. Where do most of your meals come from? Do you like to cook? Why/Why not?
   *I normally cook, but I don't like to because it takes so much time, but it is less expensive so I do it anyway.*

3. Describe briefly your weekly exercise or physical activity:

*Sit ups and push twice ups daily two sets of 20. Stretching and occasionally running*

4. How would you describe your general state of physical health? Do you suffer from any chronic disease?
   *Overall good state of health. I don't smoke, drink or do drugs.*

5. Do you have diabetes? Y X  N ____  If yes, then for how long?
   *2 Months*
   **What medications do you take and how do you monitor your dosage and blood level?**
   *Lantus 15 units and Glucophage 500mg twice daily. I check my blood sugar using freestyle test kit.*

6. What most interests you in participating in this project?
   *I was recently diagnosed with diabetes and I ate healthy, exercised regularly, and no one in my family has diabetes, yet I still have it. I would like to participate in this project because it may help me better understand this condition and maybe make others more aware of the importance of getting their levels checked and eating healthy. I hope this project will help me normalize my diabetes to a reasonable level. I was admitted into the hospital with a blood glucose level of 1200, which doctors said was the highest level they had ever seen. I was able to walk into the emergency room because I was in overall good health.*

7. What are your biggest concerns about participating in this project?
   *Will I be able to contact family and are there doctors available to speak with if any problems*

*arrive? Is the program tailored to each person or is it a broad program? How will we be compensated for participating in the documentary? How much footage is shot each day? Will I be living with others? What other productions have you completed? What other information do you have so I will know what I will be doing during the 30 days?*

8. **What are 3 things everyone knows about you?**
   *Ambitious, I am from Baltimore, and I have an entrepreneurial mind.*

9. **What are 3 things that no one knows about you? (Secret talents, private ambitions, etc.)**
   *I want to be a pilot, win an academy award, and go skydiving.*

10. **This project requires a full-time commitment for 1 month. What are the biggest obstacles to your participation in this project?**
    *I embrace all opportunities with an open mind. I figure I was given diabetes for a reason so I am trying to explore areas in which I can be an example to others who may be dealing with this as well.*

11. **Photographs:** We are interested in seeing you and your friends/family in your natural environment. Please submit some photographs that show you in your world.

**Blessings from God**

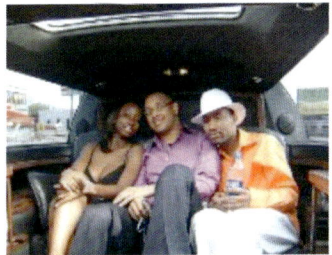 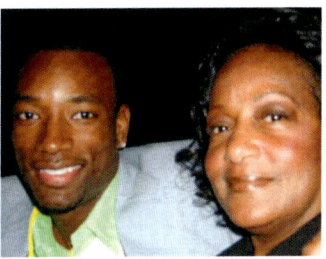

My friends: Roberta, Wayne, Ursula Clarence

Me and my cousin

12. That's it!! E-mail it to us ASAP! We look forward to meeting you!!

         Raw for 30!
         Documentary Film Project

It was a week before I heard back from the film producers. I opened up my email and saw that I was accepted as a participant in the film — one of six people chosen out of hundreds of applications. I was so happy to have received such an amazing opportunity.

# CHAPTER 6

# Experience at The Tree of Life

This experience was a new beginning that started me towards a healthier life. I had no idea what raw food was and thought we were going to be eating raw meat, but I was open to whatever it would take to reverse my diabetes. Thank goodness the diet didn't consist of raw meat. It was simply raw vegetables, nuts, and seeds — no dairy and no grains or fruits.

I had never been to the west coast, let alone Arizona. It was nothing like I had imagined. I always pictured a desert with sand blowing across it, similar to what you would see in the movies. Actually, it was pretty nice and the weather was great, with temperatures in the mid-sixties in the winter. There were cacti and trees.

I was picked up from the airport and given my first sample of raw food, which was a raw nut plate and a salad. It tasted pretty good and was filling. It took a little over an hour to drive to The Tree of Life in Patagonia, Arizona.

The Tree of Life Rejuvenation Center was rugged. There weren't any paved roads, concrete sidewalks, or exterior lights to help you see at night. The rooms were small and consisted of two beds, two nightstands, and a trashcan. The purpose of such sparse amenities is to create a peaceful environment that allows you to connect with nature. In the beginning, I had no choice but to connect with nature: I had no Internet access and my phone was always roaming. I have to admit, however, that this experience was pretty peaceful and serene.

There were six participants total: Henry, Bill, Aunt Pam, Austin, Michelle, and myself. We spent thirty days at The Tree of Life and we all became a big family. It was a fun and emotional journey as we all battled our addictions to food and our socially formed beliefs about it. Some of us were able to stick with the program, but others were unable to adhere to the strict requirements in order to reverse their diabetes.

The food was basic and didn't include many seasonings or ingredients. I quickly got over the bland taste and immediately focused on the benefits of a raw food diet. Within two weeks I was off of insulin and my blood sugar levels were normal. This change sold me on the whole experience.

I felt my life being restored. Just two months previously, it literally took me two minutes to walk up a flight of stairs. I couldn't breathe, my muscles wouldn't contract, and I would sit there leaning on the railing struggling to pull myself up the stairs. In as little as two weeks I was off medications and running up a mountain, breathing in the fresh air and feeling alive again.

After completing my thirty-day journey at The Tree of Life I felt rejuvenated, like my mind and body were in balance. I became aware of a new purpose in life: to help other people reverse diabetes. The knowledge I gained from Dr. Cousens, the doctor at The Tree of Life, reignited my passion for medicine.

# CHAPTER 7

# Experience in Naturopathic Medical School

After reversing my type 1 diabetes, I spent years interning at Johns Hopkins Hospital with some of the top cardiovascular surgeons and neurosurgeons. I enjoyed scrubbing into surgery and I even liked cath lab where we performed numerous balloon angioplasties for our heart patients. My heart had previously been set on being a cardiovascular surgeon. However, after my own recovery from diabetes, I no longer wanted to treat people only after they were sick and dying. I wanted to learn how to keep people healthy and actually help them to reverse disease.

I felt that conventional medical school would not have much to offer me since I did not want to be an Allopathic Doctor (M.D.). Instead, I started researching becoming an Osteopathic Doctor (D.O.) but soon learned that they were trained in the same way as Allopathic Doctors and practiced very similar medicine. One day I was at my friend's graduation party and someone mentioned that their doctor was a Naturopathic Doctor (N.M.D.). I had never heard of that type of doctor before. I wasn't even sure if they were real doctors. I did a lot of research and it turned out that naturopathic doctors were indeed real doctors.

Naturopathic medicine is built on the philosophical premise that disease is cured by identifying and removing the root cause. This is in contrast with the allopathic medical philosophy, taught at most medical schools and practiced by the majority of medical doctors, which relies on the concept of identifying diseases or symptoms and then prescribing drugs to manage or combat those conditions. The allopathic system considers the disease or symptom to be the actual problem, as opposed to addressing the underlying causes that produced the disease or symptom in the first place. After doing a lot of research about different schools' curriculums and the way naturopathic doctors practice medicine, I found that naturopathic doctors' ideas about health were more in line with mine.

At the time there were only five naturopathic medical schools that were accredited: University of Bridgeport College of Naturopathic Medicine, located in Bridgeport, Connecticut; National College of Natural Medicine, located in Portland, Oregon; Bastyr University, located in Seattle, Washington; Canadian College of Naturopathic Medicine, located in Toronto, Ontario, Canada; and Southwest College of Naturopathic Medicine, located in Tempe, Arizona. Currently there are seven schools, which now include National University of Health Sciences, located in Chicago, Illinois and Boucher Institute of Naturopathic Medicine, located in Vancouver, British Columbia, Canada. Choosing which school to attend was easy for me. Southwest College is the only school located in a warm climate, plus it is a two or three hour drive to The Tree of Life in Patagonia, AZ.

I started my studies at Southwest College of Naturopathic Medicine in August 2007. Orientation was inspiring because we shared our stories, our health struggles, and the health struggles of our family members that led us to naturopathic medicine. Becoming a Naturopathic Doctor felt like a calling, and we were all there because we wanted to answer the call.

The first two years of school focused on the basic sciences and the philosophy of naturopathic medicine. Our classes included subjects in biochemistry, embryology, anatomy and physiology, cell biology, immunology, genetics, botanical medicine, hydrotherapy, toxicology, pathology, physiotherapy, traditional Chinese medicine, nutrition, and homeopathy, as well as courses on how to heal oneself. It was an intense program. There were plenty of sleepless nights and lonely nights, all undertaken in an effort to gain a better understanding of how the body works and to appreciate how an imbalance in one system can lead to an imbalance in another system.

## The Raw Truth: The Recipe for Reversing Diabetes

My biggest challenge in medical school involved the nutritional courses. These courses were a bit of a struggle for me because they brought about inner conflict. The material was straightforward and easy for me to understand, but I had a hard time assimilating it into my current lifestyle. In our nutritional courses we talked about micronutrients, which include vitamins and minerals. We also discussed macronutrients, which include fats, proteins, and carbohydrates. The course covered various diets, including raw foods, Atkins, Mediterranean, and the blood type diet, to name a few.

Based on my own experience, I knew that I felt better eating a raw food diet. As we talked about the various diets, however, I began to second-guess my instincts. My blood type is O+ and on the blood type diet, it is recommended that type Os eat plenty of animal meat protein. Other discussions revealed that there are no civilizations that survive on an all-raw diet. Hearing these things was very confusing to me.

I started thinking to myself, "Well, maybe I should be eating meat." There was a part of me that wanted to do that because I really missed the taste of hamburgers, chicken, and fish. However, there was another part of me that kept thinking that this couldn't be the right choice because none of those other diets reversed diabetes. Honestly, I was a mess. I knew what I was doing was right, but the information being presented in school did not confirm my beliefs.

I caved to temptation and started eating cooked foods. The first time I bit into a hamburger, the taste was orgasmic. I could not believe how good it tasted. I found myself gorging on this food, yet I never felt satisfied; I was constantly hungry and felt tired. Eventually, my diet went from 100 percent raw to about 25 percent raw. Between December of 2007 and March of 2008, I ate chicken, pizza, hot dogs, hamburgers, fish, and chips, and drank sodas.

It was literally an addiction, and as a result, I started to feel horrible. I would never intentionally do anything intentionally that could be deadly, and I'd never done drugs because I knew how harmful they were, yet I was eating all of this dead food. I started feeling tired again, my nose was always clogged up with mucus, and my bowels were irregular. Even with all of these symptoms, I did not want to believe that the food was what was causing me so much trouble. I was denying my body and I would find myself fiending for my next fix of hot wings. My eating habits had spiraled out of control.

My blood sugar levels still stayed in the normal range until late March 2008. I had just returned from Baltimore, Maryland, and I had caught the flu and was experiencing a fever and fatigue. Not only was I sick, but my blood sugar levels were in the 200s. They hadn't been that high since January of 2006. There I was with type 1 diabetes and my antibodies working against my pancreas.

I reasoned that the flu had caused my immune system to act up, my immune system had started to destroy my pancreas, and now the diabetes was back. However, as much as I wanted to believe my theory to be true, all I kept thinking to myself was, "Oh my God, I really MESSED UP! Why did I do this to myself?" It wasn't the flu that caused the diabetes to come back. It was my actions over the previous three months.

I was scared and I could not believe I had allowed this to happen. I had known what it took to be diabetes free, but I'd thrown it all out the window because I wanted to eat foods that everyone else was eating. Honestly, I enjoyed the taste of the raw foods I prepared, and loved the fresh salads, raw pizzas, nut burgers, raw cheesecakes, and soups. Yet here I was in medical school feeling stupid because I knew exactly what it took to be healthy, yet I'd stopped doing it. You don't realize what you have until you are on the verge of losing it.

# CHAPTER 8

# Rediscovery of Raw Foods

Health is something you earn; you don't catch it. I didn't catch the flu or diabetes; I earned it. The foods I started eating weakened my body, mind, and immune system. I was looking for life while consuming death.

With my blood sugar levels in the 200s, I was once again faced with diabetes. I went to the doctor and was prescribed Lantus 15 units daily. Although I was really disappointed with myself, I knew I had to move past the disappointment. Eventually I picked myself up off the floor and remembered that I knew the recipe for reversing diabetes.

I cleaned out all the junk that filled my refrigerator and cabinets. I told myself that only healthy foods would enter my body. During this process, I also accepted the fact that I was responsible for my own health and realized that hundreds of millions of people are addicted to food. The information I was learning in school had me believing that it was acceptable to eat animals. However, when it comes to reversing diabetes, eating meat is not an option.

I had to retrain the way I thought. I could no longer accept the information I was hearing as true for me. I could no longer fool myself into believing otherwise, because there is no greater fool than a fool who fools himself. I was that fool addicted to cooked, processed foods.

Humans are the only beings who cook their food. We claim to be omnivorous, yet most of us dislike the idea of blood and the taste of meat, so we cook it until it's burnt and then disguise it with sauces, seasonings, and toppings. We eat meat because we were brought up eating meat and we were told that we have to eat meat in order to get protein. We were told that eating meat make us strong and healthy.

The belief that you cannot survive without eating meat is wrong.

Appetite is a learned behavior. My appetite was built on sugary and processed foods, so whenever I felt "hungry," I would reach for a Snickers bar because it satisfied the craving I was experiencing. In actuality, it wasn't hunger that I was experiencing, but appetite. The people truly experiencing hunger are those helpless children in impoverished countries like Africa and even right here in America who honestly have nothing to eat and whose bodies are feeding on themselves. That's hunger!

You are in a position to make choices that will feed your body, mind, and spirit. You can make a choice to eat foods that are alive and that provide you with the nutrition and minerals your body needs to survive. We don't make these choices naturally anymore because we were told that a salad isn't good enough and you need to have meat with that meal. Now, our society has reached a point where the meal is nothing but meat. I have friends who ate green vegetables twice a year at most because they believed that fast food was all the nutrition their body needed to survive. It is true, the body can survive off of that stuff, but the bigger question is for how long and at what cost.

Nature doesn't lie. When you wake up from your slumber and stop drinking fluoridated water, you will see that the recipe for healthy living has already been provided for you. The longest living organisms on the planet are those closest to the sources of life and are able to use the sun and water for energy. Those are plants, trees, algae, and bushes. Methuselah, the oldest known living tree in the world, is 4,843 years old as of 2012. When you look at nature you start to realize that the information you were told as a child does not square with your observations as an adult. Elephants are big, strong and live around eighty years on a plant-based diet. Yet dogs eat a meat-based diet and live for six to fifteen years. Not only are our pets living short lives, but they are also afflicted with the same diseases that we have: diabetes, cancer, glaucoma, and heart disease, to name a few. Maybe it's because we are eating a lot of the same processed foods.

When it comes to those processed foods, we don't really know what's in the food that we are eating. I met a lady from Thailand who told me that her family used to eat cockroaches and beetles. She even said that she occasionally missed eating them. When I shared this story with other people, almost everyone, including me, was disgusted by the thought of eating cockroaches. I used to see cockroaches around the house as a little kid and the thought of picking one up and eating it never crossed my mind. I actually recall screaming at the top of my lungs and running the other way. The big kicker, for all of us who thought eating bugs was disgusting, is that if you like Starbucks' strawberry Frappuccinos, then you have already had your fair share of insects. The manufacturer uses crushed cochineal beetles to give the drink its red color. Bon appetit!

The most interesting thing about eating processed foods is that manufacturers can hide anything they want under natural ingredients or other flavors. Recently we found out that a lot of the meats sold in grocery stores consist of a pink slime, which actually is the result of beef being treated with ammonia. I used to use ammonia to clean my floors, and the bottle clearly said, "Do not ingest. If accidentally ingested, please call poison control." Yet the Food and Drug Administration has okayed this pink slime to be sold in stores as food.

Retraining the way you think is the only way you will be able to maintain a healthy lifestyle. In today's artificial world, we have not been brought up to be healthy, yet we are being told that the way we are living is healthy and if you happen to get sick then doctors are there to fix you with drugs and surgery. Through my own experience I knew that the only way to escape chronic disease is to maintain a lifestyle based on health and not death.

I started back on my raw foods plan. Within two weeks my blood sugar level returned to normal and I was once again insulin free. I started to really appreciate the beauty and life that raw food brings. I consume about 80 to 90 percent raw foods and 10 to 20 percent cooked vegan.

When I started seeing patients as a medical student in 2009, I felt more confident in my ability to help. I honestly felt like my personal health struggles allowed me to see the struggles of my patients and I was better equipped to help them overcome their health issues. I was finally beginning to feel like I could help make a difference in my friends', family members', and patients' lives.

I was reminded that food is medicine, and as a doctor, my first choice is eating raw foods. If I didn't take responsibility of my health, I would still be taking insulin. At that point, I realized that I no longer wanted to be a part of the conventional medical model.

# CHAPTER 9

# The True Medical Model

**Insurance**

From the time of its conception, health insurance was never designed to protect your health; it was originally called sickness insurance. Sickness insurance was offered as early as 1847 by Massachusetts Health Insurance of Boston, which was the first company to offer a policy with comprehensive benefits. At that time health care was not very costly. Most services were performed in the home. Doctors would make house calls and births took place in the comfort of the home. The main cost of being sick was the wages you would lose while you were unable to work. Sickness insurance was designed to cover your wages in the event you became ill, so it was more like modern-day disability insurance than modern-day health insurance.

In the United States, the first individual "health" insurance plans became available during the Civil War. These plans were designed to provide coverage for injuries related to travel by steamboat or railway. Individual accident insurance was profitable for insurance companies. Over time these plans expanded to offer more coverage for illness and injury, which of course resulted in higher premiums for the insured. As improvements in medicines, treatments, and research made medicine more reliable, the cost of medical care increased.

Health insurance is a term that relates to a contract wherein the individual pays a regular premium with the expectation that should the individual have health problems, the insurer will provide for them. The term dates to the Progressive Era in the United States, where the debate about the role of the government in health care was already well underway. Though health insurance in America has its origins in a related system called "sickness insurance," it wasn't until the British passed their National Insurance Act in 1911, which referred to "health insurance," that the term came into favor.

In the United States, most people still felt that health insurance was not necessary and opted for sickness insurance plans instead. Health insurance did not become mainstream until around 1929, when a group of teachers in Dallas formed a partnership with a local hospital that provided a set amount of hospitalization and sick days in exchange for a fixed, prepaid fee. This time period marked a shift from getting reimbursed for lost wages due to illness to paying for being sick. Treatment now cost more than the wages people lost while ill.

Prepaid hospital services increased during the Depression because they provided a way to insure people's health during difficult economic times. The American Hospital Association (AHA) started to encourage other hospitals to develop similar plans to the one implemented in Dallas. These plans provided hospitals with a source of income even if they weren't treating patients. This created a lot of competition between hospitals to create better plans. Eventually, with the help of the AHA, many hospitals joined together and formed Blue Cross.

The Blue Cross plan benefitted hospitals but didn't offer much for individual doctors. Physicians wanted to retain more control of their patients' care and maintain a doctor-patient relationship, so they organized their own prepaid plans. This eventually led to the development of the Blue Shield plan, which not only competed with Blue Cross but also gave patients another alternative for care.

Another reason why Blue Shield was formed was that physicians were concerned that the social security legislation being passed at that time would lead to heavily regulated, compulsory health insurance that would devastate patient choice and doctor-patient relationships. With the Blue Shield plan, physicians were able to price discriminate and charge patients the difference between what the physician received from the insurance company and the actual cost of service.

Nationalized health insurance ceased to be a possibility in 1965, when Congress enacted Medicare and Medicaid. Medicare provided essential hospital insurance and subsidized medical insurance for people over sixty-five. Medicaid provided care for low-income people, though the federal-state program varied across state lines according to each state's relative per-capita income.

By the 1970s, the United States federal government conducted studies to determine which groups of Americans were most likely to be uninsured. They found that the majority of the uninsured lived in poverty or near the poverty line, and many of those were children. This discovery led to the creation of child-specific health programs and expanded Medicaid. These child-specific health programs and expanded Medicaid have been somewhat successful in providing care to those needing it, yet the number of uninsured Americans still rose, and rose at a greater rate within the middle class.

In 1996, Congress passed two bills in an attempt to show the American people that the federal government was committed to regulating the health insurance industry. The Mental Health Parity Act increased psychiatric benefits by mandating that, among group plans that offer mental health coverage, the limits for mental health coverage be no less than the limits for physical illnesses. The Health Insurance Portability and Accountability Act (HIPAA) brought about important medical legislation, including helping employees maintain insurance when they were between jobs, became self-employed, or were otherwise separated from an employer-packaged managed health care plan. The bill came three years after Congress rejected President Bill Clinton's plan that would have provided health insurance for all Americans. HIPAA did, however, allow the federal government to join states in overseeing and regulating the health insurance industry.

The biggest problem with health insurance is that it is a business. The only way a business can stay in business is if it makes money. The only way a health insurance company can make money is by taking in more than they spend. This means higher premiums and less payment to doctors or less care for patients. The current U.S. healthcare system is tragically corrupt and dysfunctional. The structure of the system violates fundamental insurance risk principles and has inherent

## The True Medical Model

conflicts of interest that prevent quality national health care delivery and cost efficiency.

Health care rationing by insurance companies is the direct result of a conflict of interest between providing insurance benefits to paying members in need of health care and earning profits for corporate shareholders. Insurance company employees are paid bonuses based on how little care they approve. Companies have denial and delay procedures that cause suffering and death.

The truth is that no one would buy health insurance if they didn't feel a need for health insurance. The need has been created because people constantly see their family and friends become sick. If you believe that I will be sick one day, then you will believe that I need health insurance to protect me when I become ill.

The other reason why people buy health insurance is the cost of medical care. People buy insurance when the cost of care is so high that you would not be able to afford it without health insurance. We can see this daily; it's common for people to lose their homes or file for bankruptcy because of medical expenses. At least 60% of U.S. personal bankruptcies are due to medical bills. Of these, 68% of the bankruptcy filers had health insurance but could not cover the deductibles, co-pays, and treatment denials, or they became so sick that they lost their jobs and their insurance. It is a shame that you have to choose between your house and your life.

The term should be changed from "health insurance" to "body warranty" or back to "sickness insurance" because health insurance is not geared towards health. Just like a car warranty, the bulk of the payments you make will only help you once your body breaks down and you get sick. Someone with heart disease can expect their health care costs will be upwards of one million dollars. We already know that it is cheaper to prevent a problem than to try to repair it.

There is very little coverage that goes towards keeping your body operating like a well-oiled machine. We know that the keys to health are exercise, diet, sleep, rest, relaxation, and love. Health insurance provides very little assistance with any of those things unless you have developed a problem. The way to be healthy, however, is to take steps to keep problems from ever arising. Health insurance should cover gym membership and provide discounts for healthy food, vacations, and outings with family and friends. That's how you ensure health. The likelihood of the system changing in this way is probably the same as the odds of getting struck by lightening three times on the same day. So clearly, taking care of your health is up to you.

## Food

Now that you have health insurance, let's create the diseases that make it worth having. The top health conditions that are fatal in the U.S., including heart disease, cancer, stroke, obesity, and diabetes, are caused by lifestyle choices. These conditions are heavily driven by agribusiness and food corporations, who push and advertise terrible health choices, even targeting children to get them started down an unhealthy path. The food choices you and your family make are the reason why we believe we should be paying for health insurance.

It is apparent that food can either heal us or kill us. If you have seen the documentary film Super Size Me, in which Morgan Spurlock ate McDonald's for every meal for 30 days, you saw how his health began to deteriorate in only that short period of time. On the opposite end of the spectrum, if you saw my film Simply Raw: Reversing Diabetes in 30 Days, you saw people regaining their health in 30 days. Food is medicine.

Food is a multi-billion dollar industry that uses a lot of its resources for advertising. Agribusiness and food corporations spend a lot of money to convince us that their food is good for us and our bodies. Cow's milk is one ideal example of this dynamic. Several decades ago, the advertisements for cow's milk were so convincing that people began believing that there was no better product than cow's milk. Mothers would stop breastfeeding and opt for formula or cow's milk instead.

This was a big change from most of human history, when the

consumption of cow's milk was very low. Cow's milk was indeed mass-produced from the early 1800s to around 1917, but production was plagued with problems. Milk consumption was linked to illness and diseases such as typhoid and tuberculosis.

This production problem was resolved after Louis Pasteur, considered one of the fathers of microbiology, studied milk in order to prove his "germ theory," which stated that infectious diseases and food-borne illnesses were caused by germs. Pasteur's research demonstrated that harmful microbes in milk and wine caused sickness, and he invented a process — now called "pasteurization" — whereby the liquids were rapidly heated and cooled to kill most of the organisms. This technique, made mandatory in 1917, is what allowed for the increased consumption of milk. So thanks to Pasteur, we can now drink milk and not get sick and die immediately; instead, it takes a little more time.

The milkman appeared around the 1920s and would deliver milk to homes two or three times per week. The milk that most Americans consumed came from local farms, but as the process of mass production of milk improved, so did the consumption. Milk consumption increased greatly in 1940 after legislation was enacted to provide federal assistance for distributing milk to schoolchildren in Chicago. By 1946 the National School Lunch Act passed, mandating that each lunch include between one-half and two pints of whole milk. By the 1950s, almost all households were consuming milk on a daily basis. Coincidentally, cancer rates also increased during this time and peaked around the 1970s.

The consumption of milk has never been of great benefit to humans. Research shows that type 1 diabetes has a strong correlation to early consumption of cow's milk. As children, we were told to drink cow's milk because it is high in calcium and prevents osteoporosis, but in actuality, cow's milk is acidic and causes loss of calcium from the bones. What we have learned from the China Study by T. Collin Campbell is that consumption of the protein casein, which is found in dairy, promotes cancer.

Another major cause of disease is consuming dead animal flesh. When

**The Raw Truth: The Recipe for Reversing Diabetes**

I go and speak, I ask audience members why they eat meat. Children as young as nine years old answer, "Because we need protein." We can thank the meat industry for making us believe that if we did not eat meat we would not get protein. It is clear that we need protein for survival; however, the source of protein has an even greater impact on life. In nature, cows, elephants, giraffes, and a host of other vegetarian animals are able to eat plant material and convert it into protein. At some point in history, the notion came about that humans were not a part of the animal kingdom and were unable to do the same.

Originally Americans ate grass fed beef. Raised on pasture, cattle reared before the 1950s usually took two or three years to be ready for the slaughterhouse. Steers were fed grain occasionally and in small quantities, and farmers tended to use corn as a supplement rather than a staple of their livestock's diets.

After World War II, production of corn increased and the economic boom of the 1950s prompted higher consumer demand for meat. Farmers and ranchers began feeding their cattle corn to increase their size and make them fatter. Because of the surplus of corn, it was cheaper and more efficient than grass. Feeding cattle corn enabled them to be brought to market in as few as fifteen months. Moreover, it allowed farmers to feed cattle in confined pens or lots, reducing ranchers' land costs and limiting their risk of losing livestock to predators and bad weather.

With cheaper feed in the equation, beef prices fell, and Americans began to purchase more and more beef, most of it corn-fed. By 1960, Americans ate a yearly average of more than 66 pounds of beef each. By 1975, that number had grown to 88.5 pounds of beef per person per year. With all the research that has been coming out showing the harmful effects of red meat, consumption declined to 66.1 pounds of beef per person per year in 2004. However, the consumption of other meats such as chicken tripled from 20.5 pounds per person per year in the 1950s to 66.5 pounds per person per year in 2004. As the consumption of meat increased, so did the rates of heart disease, cancer, and diabetes.

Americans have a huge sweet tooth and consume too much sugar and sweet-tasting foods and beverages. In 2000, each American consumed an average of 152 pounds of caloric sweeteners per person per year. That amounted to more than two-fifths of a pound or 52 teaspoonfuls of added sugars per person per day in 2000.

Sugar consumption has a huge impact on the body. Sugar raises your insulin levels, which causes you to store excess glucose as fat, which leads to obesity. It also inhibits the release of growth hormones, which in turn depresses the immune system. Sugar also fuels cancer. Cancer cells have seventeen times more insulin receptors than a normal cell. They can only survive by taking in glucose to use for energy. If you are consuming large amounts of sugar and have cancer, then you are giving the cancer what it needs to live. You have to realize that food isn't just food; it may be a business to some, but for you, it is the key to your health.

This is your chance to wake up and stop believing the stuff they are feeding you is actually good for you. It is one thing to eat something because it tastes good, but it is another issue to eat something and believe it is good for you when it really isn't. You can clearly see how the foods people eat are making them sick, so people then feel like they must get health insurance. And if you are sick, then the conventional medical system has a way to make you feel like you are getting better, even though you are not.

## Pharmaceuticals

In nineteenth century, pneumonia and influenza were the leading causes of death in the United States, followed by tuberculosis and diarrhea. Physicians had few weapons in their arsenal to fight disease. Often they were left helpless as patients lay feverish and tossing on the bed and then slipped away.

Louis Pasteur began investigating anthrax in 1879. France and some other parts of Europe were suffering from an anthrax epidemic that had killed a large number of sheep, and the disease was attacking humans as well. German physician Robert Koch announced the isolation of the anthrax bacillus, which Pasteur confirmed. Koch and Pasteur independently provided definitive experimental evidence that the anthrax bacillus was indeed responsible for the infection. This firmly established the germ theory of disease, which then emerged as the fundamental concept underlying medical microbiology.

Pasteur wanted to apply the principle of vaccination to anthrax. After determining the conditions that led to the organism's loss of virulence, he prepared attenuated cultures of the bacillus. In the spring of 1881 he obtained financial support, mostly from farmers, to conduct a large-scale public experiment to test anthrax immunization. The experiment took place in Pouilly-le-Fort, located on the southern outskirts of Paris. Pasteur immunized 70 farm animals, giving them two inoculations with vaccines of different potencies at intervals of twelve days. A vaccine from a low-virulence culture was given to half the sheep and was followed by a second vaccine from a more virulent culture. Two weeks after these initial inoculations, both the vaccinated and control sheep were inoculated with a virulent strain of anthrax. Within a few days, all the control sheep died, whereas all the vaccinated animals survived. The experiment was a complete success and its results validated the work of Louis Pasteur.

As more vaccine discoveries were made, pharmaceutical companies rose to the task of developing these compounds, ensuring safety and efficacy and mass-producing and marketing the medicines. This is well illustrated by the discovery and development of insulin. Until the late nineteenth century, diabetes mellitus meant death. At that time, scientists figured out that the disease is caused by a malfunctioning pancreas that fails to produce insulin, and attempted to isolate the hormone. All experiments failed until 1921, when Canadian physician Frederick Banting isolated the hormone. Banting, Macleod, and the rest of the team patented their insulin extract but gave away all their rights to the University of Toronto. Very soon after the discovery of insulin, the medical firm Eli Lilly started large-scale production of the extract. As early as 1923, the firm was producing enough insulin to supply the world.

Although insulin doesn't cure diabetes, it represented one of the biggest discoveries in medicine and seemed like a miracle. People with diabetes so severe that they had only days left to live were saved. And as long as they kept getting their insulin, they could live an almost normal life.

In the past hundred years, pharmaceutical research has helped transform health care from a largely palliative practice to a science-based endeavor. Due in part to this transformation and in part to improvements in sanitation, average life expectancy in the U.S. has increased from 47 years in 1900 to more than 78.5 years in 2009.

In the past, drugs were made to address the underlying cause of disease, which at the time was usually due to infectious agents. The problem with contemporary pharmaceutical drugs is that they are not intended to provide a cure. They are designed to deal with the symptom, and not the cause, of disease. The cause of high blood pressure is not high blood pressure, so a drug that lowers your high blood pressure does not solve the problem.

We can no longer expect pharmaceutical drugs to solve the problems created by lifestyle choices. If you do not change your lifestyle, then one pharmaceutical drug will lead to more. Nowadays, it's quite possible for people to be on 15 or 20 pharmaceutical drugs without getting better. In the beginning they may think they are getting better, but over time their health becomes progressively worse. Now we have to look at the people giving us this false sense of security.

## Doctors

Throughout the history of medicine, the role, status, and required qualifications of a doctor have changed. At various times doctors have been gods, priests, or scientists, or even viewed as a waste of money or the agents of death. Doctors have relied on prayer, herbal potions, observation, cleanliness, or scientific knowledge to treat or prevent illness, with varying success. Although today certain treatments seem guaranteed to shorten rather than prolong life, the common aim of all doctors throughout the history of medicine has been to cure their patients.

## The Raw Truth: The Recipe for Reversing Diabetes

The first doctors were the shamans or medicine men who practiced the prehistoric medicine of the Stone Age. Medicine men combined the worlds of religion and rational medicine. They used some rational or practical techniques, such as setting broken bones in clay or using herbal remedies made from local plants such as coca or orchid bulbs. At the same time they used religious rituals to treat any illness that they could not understand. Religious ceremonies and techniques such as trepanning (drilling a hole in the skull) were used to drive away the evil spirit causing the illness. Skills were handed down by example and word of mouth since there were no schools or written language to spread information. Medicine men were accepted as doctors because they were the closest people in the tribe to the gods and gained their powers of healing from their deities.

Imhotep was an imaginative Egyptian architect who is also venerated as the first medical professor and founder of a medical school that promoted a safe, calm, and disciplined environment in which students could discover and develop their talents. He diagnosed and treated hundreds of diseases including diseases of the abdomen, bladder, rectum, and eyes, and many of the skin, hair, nails and tongue. He treated tuberculosis, gallstones, appendicitis, gout, and arthritis.

Very significant resources still used in today's modern medical practices trace their origins to Imhotep's medical school: medical tools that we recognize such as forceps, scissors, and surgical blades were all designed in imitation of ancient Egyptian medical apparatus. And certain remedies for elementary disorders first utilized in ancient Egyptian medicine are still practiced today. Castor oil as a laxative, honey as an antimicrobial, and Acacia as a cough remedy all result from Imhotep's teachings and forward-thinking medical protocols.

In ancient Greek medicine, doctors were able to build on the ideas of Egyptians such as Imhotep by taking a more philosophical approach to knowledge. Greek doctors continued to practice both spiritual and rational forms of medicine, but there was more separation between these two traditions. The most influential Greek doctor was Hippocrates, who practiced in the fifth and fourth centuries BC. He believed that illness was not caused by the gods but was the result of the body's elements being out of balance with the environment. Hippocrates believed that food was a good source of healing. His most quoted phrase is, "Let food be thy medicine and medicine be thy food."

The role, status, beliefs, and abilities of doctors have changed over the thousands of years since the Stone Age. Spiritual explanations for illness and disease have declined in importance, to be replaced by practical and rational medicine. Doctors have ceased to be priests, and the science of medicine has become all-powerful. Although herbal remedies have remained in use throughout the history of medicine, the medical understanding of why certain herbs work has changed. The ideas of certain doctors such as Galen remained dominant for long periods, and the discoveries of others, such as Vesalius and Pasteur, have revolutionized medical practice. What remains true of the profession, however, from the prehistoric medicine man to the modern scientific specialist of today, is that a doctor's job is to cure their patients using any available knowledge and permissible technique.

Doctors use whatever resources they have available to diagnose, prevent, and cure disease. Pharmaceutical medicine became popular after the discovery of penicillin because it gave us hope that we could eradicate the most common fatal diseases, such as smallpox, typhoid fever, and bubonic plague, which at the time were caused by pathogens. However, in our present-day society, we are relying on pharmaceutical drugs to cure diseases such as heart disease, cancer, and diabetes, which are all caused by lifestyle choices. Today's doctors need to use different resources to solve today's health problems. You also have to remember that we are responsible for our own health. Wake up, people: if you want health, you have to earn it.

# CHAPTER 10

# Escaping the Health Care Model

I f you are diabetic and are ready to change your life to address the root, and not just the symptoms, of your disease, then here are some first steps that you can take to get started.

Meet with your doctor to have a physical exam, have blood drawn, and discuss the lab results with him or her. The labs to have drawn are Complete Blood Count (CBC), CMP, Ha1C, Fasting insulin, C-peptide, Lipid Panel, c-reactive protein, Vitamin D 25-OH, Iron, Ferritin, and thyroid function test. This test will give you a good understanding of your current health status.

**CBC**
The CBC is a very common test. Many patients will have baseline CBC tests done to help determine their general health status. If you are having symptoms like fatigue or weakness or if you have an infection, inflammation, bruising, or bleeding, then a CBC may be ordered to help diagnose the cause.

The test measures the levels of white blood cells, red blood cells, and platelets in the blood. Significant increases in WBCs (White Blood Cells) may help confirm that an infection is present and suggest the need for further testing to identify its cause. Decreases in the number of RBCs (anemia) can be further evaluated by looking for any changes in size or shape of the RBCs to help determine if the cause might be decreased production, increased loss, or increased destruction of RBCs. A platelet count that is low or extremely high may confirm the cause of excessive bleeding or clotting and can also be associated with diseases of the bone marrow such as leukemia.

## CMP

The Comprehensive Metabolic Panel (CMP) is a frequently ordered panel of tests that gives your doctor important information about the current status of your kidneys, liver, and electrolyte and acid/base balance, as well as providing information about your blood sugar and blood proteins. Abnormal results, and especially combinations of abnormal results, can indicate a problem that needs to be addressed.

## Ha1C

This test is used to monitor your diabetes and to aid in treatment decisions. The chart below uses the HbA1C. value to show you the average level of your blood sugar over a three-month period. Your goal is to have an HbA1C. level of 6 or below — in the green zone on the chart. If you are in the yellow to red zone, then it means your blood sugar levels are not well controlled and you are at increased risk of diabetes related complications. If your HbA1C. is really high, do not feel discouraged. My HbA1C. was 11.5 when I was first diagnosed with diabetes and it came down to 6.1 after three months on a raw food diet.

| HbA1c | 4.0 | 4.1 | 4.2 | 4.3 | 4.4 | 4.5 | 4.6 | 4.7 | 4.8 | 4.9 |
|---|---|---|---|---|---|---|---|---|---|---|
| mg/dl | 65 | 69 | 72 | 76 | 79 | 83 | 86 | 90 | 93 | 97 |
| mmol/l | 3.6 | 3.8 | 4.0 | 4.2 | 4.4 | 4.6 | 4.8 | 5.0 | 5.2 | 5.4 |
| HbA1c | 5.0 | 5.1 | 5.2 | 5.3 | 5.4 | 5.5 | 5.6 | 5.7 | 5.8 | 5.9 |
| mg/dl | 101 | 104 | 108 | 111 | 115 | 118 | 122 | 126 | 129 | 133 |
| mmol/l | 5.6 | 5.8 | 6.0 | 6.2 | 6.4 | 6.6 | 6.8 | 7.0 | 7.2 | 7.4 |
| HbA1c | 6.0 | 6.1 | 6.2 | 6.3 | 6.4 | 6.5 | 6.6 | 6.7 | 6.8 | 6.9 |
| mg/dl | 136 | 140 | 143 | 147 | 151 | 154 | 158 | 161 | 165 | 168 |
| mmol/l | 7.6 | 7.8 | 8.0 | 8.2 | 8.4 | 8.6 | 8.8 | 9.0 | 9.2 | 9.4 |

**The Raw Truth: The Recipe for Reversing Diabetes**

| HbA1c | 7.0 | 7.1 | 7.2 | 7.3 | 7.4 | 7.5 | 7.6 | 7.7 | 7.8 | 7.9 |
|---|---|---|---|---|---|---|---|---|---|---|
| mg/dl | 172 | 176 | 180 | 183 | 186 | 190 | 193 | 197 | 200 | 204 |
| mmol/l | 9.6 | 9.8 | 10.0 | 10.2 | 10.4 | 10.6 | 10.8 | 11.0 | 11.2 | 11.4 |
| HbA1c | 8.0 | 8.1 | 8.2 | 8.3 | 8.4 | 8.5 | 8.6 | 8.7 | 8.8 | 8.9 |
| mg/dl | 207 | 211 | 215 | 218 | 222 | 225 | 229 | 232 | 236 | 240 |
| mmol/l | 11.6 | 11.8 | 12.0 | 12.2 | 12.4 | 12.6 | 12.8 | 13.0 | 13.2 | 13.4 |
| HbA1c | 9.0 | 9.5 | 10.0 | 10.5 | 11.0 | 11.5 | 12.0 | 12.5 | 13.0 | 13.5 |
| mg/dl | 243 | 261 | 279 | 297 | 314 | 332 | 298 | 368 | 386 | 403 |
| mmol/l | 13.6 | 14.6 | 15.6 | 16.8 | 17.6 | 18.6 | 19.6 | 20.6 | 21.6 | 22.6 |

Note: The table to convert Hb-A1C. to Mean Plasma Glucose (MPG) is based on the following formulas:

HbA1c = (Mean Plasma Glucose mg/dl + 77.3) / 35.6
HbA1c = (Mean Plasma Glucose mmol/l + 4.29) / 1.98

Mean Plasma Glucose mg/dl = (HbA1C. x 35.6) - 77.3)
Mean Plasma Glucose mmol/dl = (HbA1C. x 1.98) - 4.29

## Fasting Insulin and C-peptide

These tests are used to determine how much insulin your body is producing and can be used to distinguish type 2 diabetes, which typically has high insulin and C-peptide levels, from type 1 diabetes, which typically has low insulin and c-peptide levels.

## Lipid Panel and C-reactive Protein

These tests are used to determine the risk of coronary heart disease. They have been shown to be good indicators of whether someone is likely to have a heart attack or stroke caused by blockage of blood vessels or hardening of the arteries (atherosclerosis).

## 1, 25-dihydroxyvitamin D

This test is used to assess your vitamin D levels. Low vitamin D levels have been linked to conditions ranging from autoimmune disorders to cancer. Ideal vitamin D levels are between 60-80 mg/ml.

## Iron and Ferritin

This test is used to assess how much iron you have in your body. Low iron levels can lead to fatigue.

## Thyroid TSH, FT3, and FT4

These tests check how well your thyroid is functioning. The hormones measured in the test regulate serotonin and norepinephrine levels in the brain. In addition, thyroid T3, T4 and other hormones are used to stimulate and regulate your metabolism. The T3 hormone is considered more metabolically active than T4.

## Support System

You are about to embark on a life-changing journey to restore your health and redefine eating. You have to commit and know that changing your diet will improve your health and reverse your diabetes. You have to look at this as a chance to save your life. It is great to have the support of friends and family members, but you have to be the one to do the work even when those around you are not able to give you direct support.

You are dealing with one of the most severe chronic diseases and it is highly affected by the foods you eat. If you live alone, you have to start off by clearing all non-healing foods out of house. No dairy, grains, breads, processed foods, fruits, meats, or pre-packaged foods. You will require only fresh vegetables, nuts, and seeds. Yes, fruit is usually good for the body, but it is not good for someone with diabetes.

If you live with family or friends, let them know that you are about to make a dramatic change in your diet and life, you are doing everything you can to beat diabetes, and you need their support. Ask them not to bring harmful foods into the house during this time period and to avoid eating around you. Of course, this is difficult because a lot of social interactions are centered on eating. You have to do this because this is your equivalent of drug rehab; your drug is food.

**The Raw Truth: The Recipe for Reversing Diabetes**

This diet isn't simply going to help you lose weight and tone up. It is supposed to save your life and restore your health. You have to constantly remind yourself of how important these changes are going to be for you.

## Starting Your Diet

Go grocery shopping before you start your diet. Make sure you have the food you need as well as plenty of options for diet friendly snacks and drinks. If you have to run out to the grocery store when you're hungry, you increase the chance of buying foods that are not diet friendly.

Pick a start date for your diet that you will stick to, and commit to that date. Some people do better starting a diet on a Monday, the beginning of the month, or some other significant date. If you're one of these people, don't be afraid to wait a few days to start. If you are gung-ho to get started, that's fine too, but do make the commitment that once you start, you will remain on the diet for at least thirty days. This will give you time to see the effects of the diet on your blood sugar levels. Go out the night before and indulge in your favorite foods. You can enjoy the taste, but know that those foods may not be healing for your body.

Talk with you doctor to see how often you should return to check your progress. It is good to monitor your blood sugar levels three times per day: once upon waking, which is called fasting glucose, again two hours after eating a meal, and a final time before bed.

## Adjusting Medications

The goal is to get you to be medication free with normal blood glucose levels. Be sure to discuss this with your doctor. At some point you are going to have to stop taking medications and allow your body to heal on its own. This is a delicate process and requires the supervision of a trained physician.

You will notice that your daily intake of insulin will decrease tremendously when you're on the raw food diet. It is important to monitor your glucose levels and the amount of insulin you take. Talk with your doctor about the best ways to reduce your insulin dosages while on the diet. If you are on a fast acting insulin, then talk with your doctor about discontinuing your fast acting insulin and replacing it with a long acting insulin such as Lantus.

Fast acting insulin quickly takes glucose out of circulation, delivers it to cells, and stores the rest as fat. The problem with fast acting insulin is that it wears off quickly as well, so the glucose that was stored as fat quickly re-enters circulation. Fast acting insulin is designed to help stabilize your blood sugar levels after meals, but the foods you are eating on a raw food diet will help to stabilize your blood sugar levels naturally. You will not have the constant highs and lows, so you will no longer need fast acting insulin.

The goal is to eventually get you to a point where you and your doctor are comfortable with you no longer taking insulin. You should start off by decreasing your insulin by one-third of your usual amount: i.e., if you usually take 15 units, then you would reduce it to 10 units per day.

When you first discontinue your medications, your fasting blood sugar levels may consistently be around 200 mg/dl daily for the first week or two but will start to drop below 200 mg/dl around the third week. Over the course of six to eight weeks your fasting glucose levels should be down to 150 mg/dl without insulin and eventually return to below 100 mg/dl within three months after starting the program. Even if you are not taking any medications for your diabetes, you should still follow up with a doctor to monitor your progress.

Some people may be turned off by the three-month time frame. If you are feeling this way, then you have to realize it is only a quarter of a year. Three months goes by very fast, and typically by the third week the new diet becomes second nature. You have to once again value your life and feel that it is worth your time and effort. You can't beat diabetes unless you try.

A non-diabetic usually produces around 35 units of insulin per day and maintains an average glucose level of 85mg/dl. If you are taking more

## The Raw Truth: The Recipe for Reversing Diabetes

than 35 units of insulin per day and your blood sugar levels are not in a normal range, it is likely you have developed insulin resistance as well, and your blood glucose regulation is completely out of balance.

If you are a type 1 diabetic and have insulin resistance, your body is not producing enough insulin to maintain normal glucose levels. In addition, you are taking in too much insulin, so your body down regulates the number of insulin receptors it has on its cell surfaces, thus causing you to have elevated blood sugar levels.

If you are a type 2 diabetic with insulin resistance, your body is producing a lot of insulin, probably because your diet is stimulating your pancreas to produce it. However, if your body is constantly producing high amounts of insulin, your cells also down regulate the number of insulin receptors on their surfaces, thus causing you to have elevated blood sugar levels. For both type 1 and type 2 diabetics, if your diet is filled with processed foods, then those unhealthy fats change the fluidity of your cell membranes and insulin receptors. The receptors become less sensitive to insulin, and this also contributes to high blood sugar levels.

# CHAPTER 11

# Detoxification

The body is very effective at restoring balance and healing itself. Recall the last time you cut your finger. When you left it alone and allowed the body to work, it healed itself in a couple of weeks. Reversing diabetes works on the same principle.

Right now your body is full of toxins that need to be eliminated. This toxic buildup is an obstacle to curing disease. Elimination is just as essential as diet, which is why detoxification, the process of eliminating toxins from the body, is important.

More and more people have become aware of the affects of toxicity on their health. We have created stronger chemicals that have polluted our air, food, and water. We ingest new chemicals, use more drugs of all kinds, eat more sugar and refined foods, and abuse ourselves with various stimulants and sedatives. The incidence of many diseases has increased as well. Cardiovascular diseases, cancer, and diabetes are a few of those diseases. You can also add arthritis, allergies, obesity, and various skin problems to the list. In addition, a wide range of symptoms, such as headaches, fatigue, pains, coughs, gastrointestinal problems, and problems from immune weakness can all be related to toxicity.

A toxin is basically any substance that creates irritating and/or harmful effects in the body, undermining our health or stressing our biochemical or organ functions. This may result from medical or recreational drugs, which have side effects, or from patterns of physiology that are different from our usual functioning. Free radicals are toxins that irritate, inflame, age, and cause degeneration of body tissues. Negative psychic and spiritual influences, thought patterns, and negative emotions all can be toxins as well because they can act as stressors, change the normal physiology of the body, and possibly produce specific symptoms.

**The Raw Truth: The Recipe for Reversing Diabetes**

Toxicity occurs in our body when we take in more of any given substance than we can utilize and eliminate. Homeostasis, meaning a state in which our body functions are in balance, is disturbed when we feed ourselves more than we need or partake of specific substances that are toxic. Toxicity may depend on the dosage, frequency, or potency of the toxin. A toxin may produce an immediate or rapid onset of symptoms, as many pesticides and some drugs do; possibly, even more commonly, it may cause some long-term negative effect, such as asbestos exposure leading to lung cancer.

Toxicity occurs on two basic levels — external and internal. We can acquire toxins from our environment by breathing them, by ingesting them, or through physical contact with them. We all are exposed to toxins daily. We eat and drink them and impose them upon ourselves repeatedly and regularly. Most drugs, food additives, and allergens can create toxic elements in the body. In fact, any substance can have toxicity — water, potassium, and almost all nutrients can be a problem in certain circumstances.

On the internal level, our body produces toxins through its normal everyday functions. Biochemical, cellular, and bodily activities generate substances that need to be eliminated. The immune system, environmental factors such as pollution, radiation, cigarette smoke, and herbicides can also spawn free radicals. When these toxic substances and molecules are not eliminated, they can cause irritation or inflammation of the cells and tissues, blocking normal functions on a cellular, organ, and whole-body level. Microbes of all kinds, intestinal bacteria, foreign bacteria, yeasts, and parasites all produce metabolic waste products that we must handle. Our thoughts, emotions, and stress itself generate increased biochemical toxicity.

Properly eliminating these toxins is essential for good health. Clearly, a normally functioning body was created to handle certain levels of toxins. If our body is working well, with good immune and eliminative functions, we can handle our basic everyday exposure. The concern is with excess intake or production of toxins or a reduction in the processes of elimination. Through detoxification, we clear and filter toxins and wastes and allow our bodies to work on enhancing their basic functions.

There are three main modes of detoxification: urinary, fecal, and sweat. Our body handles toxins by neutralizing, transforming, or eliminating them. The liver helps transform many toxic substances into harmless agents, while the blood carries wastes to the kidneys; it also dumps wastes through the bile into the intestines, where much waste is eliminated. We also clear toxins when we sweat due to exercise or heat. Our sinuses and skin may also be accessory elimination organs whereby excess mucus or toxins can be released, as with sinus congestion or skin rashes, respectively.

Detoxification occurs on many levels: physically, mentally, emotionally, and spiritually. Physically, it can help clear congestion, illnesses, and disease potential. It can improve energy. Detoxifying can help rejuvenate us and prevent degeneration. Mentally, cleansing our minds of negative thought patterns is essential to health; physical detoxification aids in mental detoxification, so you will notice that your mental clarity will improve on a raw foods diet. Emotionally, detoxification helps us uncover and express feelings, especially hidden frustrations, anger, resentments, or fear, and replace them with forgiveness, love, joy, and hope. On a spiritual level, many people experience new clarity and/or an enhancement of their purpose in life during cleansing processes. By eliminating abusive habits and eating a better diet, you will be committing to a longer process and making a deeper commitment to a new way of life that will help you to really change.

Detoxification, then, is part of a transformational medicine that instills change on many levels, and this change and evolution are keys to healing. Enhancing elimination helps us deal with and clear problems from our past, from childhood and parental patterns to recent job or relationship stress. When our body has eliminated much of its toxic buildup, we feel lighter and are able to really experience the moment and be open to the future.

Detoxification is a relative term. Anything that supports our elimination can be said to help us detoxify. Your goal is to drink half of your body weight in ounces of purified water every day (i.e. a 120-pound person should drink at least 60 ounces of water). Add an additional eight ounces of water if you are pregnant. Doing this will increase your body's hydration and also help eliminate toxins through the urinary system. By eating organic, raw vegetables, you reduce the amount of toxins you are ingesting and the increased fiber increases the amount of toxins you are eliminating. You can increase your body's ability to detoxify by performing coffee enemas, which stimulate liver detoxification, and colonics, which increase the release of feces from the colon.

As you begin your detoxification process or "detox," you may experience both physical and mental symptoms. These symptoms appear when you alter your life by changing your diet, exercising, or discontinuing a current habit like smoking. These symptoms include headache, stomachache, cough, diarrhea, skin eruptions (rash), clogged sinuses, and fever, as well as feeling run-down and irritable. The symptoms may be of short duration and be a slight irritation, or they could last longer and cause you considerable discomfort.

The most concerning question I receive from people who have switched to a raw foods diet is about the increased frequency of diarrhea. I ensure them that this is a normal occurrence and it is the body's attempt to finally get rid of all the toxins from the foods that had been stored in the colon. After you have finished using the bathroom, get up and look into the toilet. Is there anything in there that you want to take back? The diarrhea isn't a result of the raw vegetables being bad for the body, but the body finally waking up from its slumber to get the crap out.

Being afraid of the detox process can result feeling like you are doing something wrong. However, this is a misunderstanding. You have to look at it from the perspective that cooked food is a drug and you are detoxing from it the same way that a heroin addict has to detox. Yes, the heroin addict feels better on the drug, but it is indeed killing them. They only later realize how amazing they really feel once they have been away from drugs for quite some time. Understanding this apparent contradiction is perhaps the first, and most important, hurdle you must get over when making a dietary or lifestyle change.

Most detox symptoms last from four to eight days. It is important to remind yourself that you have to move past the way you are feeling at the moment and know that you will start to feel better in a few days. To decrease detox symptoms, drink plenty of water and make sure your bowels are eliminating properly. The large intestine is five feet long, so if you are eating three times per day and not eliminating three times per day than you are indeed constipated. The longer the feces sit there, the more chances there are for toxins to recirculate. Do not resort to your old habits and begin eating cooked foods to make yourself feel better.

# CHAPTER 12

# Supplements

Your main goal is to be healthy. The raw food diet will fill all of your nutritional needs, but you are currently in a weakened state of health and require a little extra help to restore your body to optimal condition. There are supplements that can help you get back into balance more quickly. The goal is to use supplements to restore health. Then, you can allow nature to maintain it without the need of as much supplementation. Some of these vitamins you may not need to supplement, and most others can be found in a good multivitamin. Talk with your doctor to found out the right supplements for you.

**Vitamin C**
Vitamin C. is a water-soluble vitamin that must be replenished each day. The body absorbs as much as it needs, and the amount it needs depends on the health of the individual. A person who has an illness, such as a cold, will require higher levels of vitamin C. and the body will absorb more of it than in a healthy person. (For example, a healthy person's normal absorption may be 50% of 2 grams of vitamin C. When the person develops a cold, their body could absorb as much of 100% of 2 grams of vitamin C. and may still require more.) You will know your upper limit of vitamin C. by your bowel tolerance. Too much vitamin C. will typically result in diarrhea.

Some of the benefits of Vitamin C. are that it boosts the immune system, helps repair wounds, and restores collagen. It also reduces the risk of developing diabetes. When coupled with vitamin E, it helps get sugar out of the bloodstream and into the cells. As much as 50% of vitamin C. is lost when you cook foods containing it.

Dosage: 2 gram (2,000 mg) per day, and you can increase it to bowel tolerance.

## Vitamin D

Our body is capable of producing its own vitamin D via exposure to the sun. The best way to produce vitamin D is by going outside with mostly exposed skin between the hours of 10 a.m. and 2 p.m. with little cloud cover. The exposure time is 10-20 minutes in people with low pigmentation and up to 60-80 minutes for people with higher pigmentation. Unfortunately for many Americans, it is difficult to obtain the required amount of daily sun exposure to produce adequate amounts of vitamin D.

Vitamin D provides protection against diabetes mellitus, autoimmune disorders, osteoporosis, and cancers of the breast, colon, uterus, and prostate. It strengthens bones and reduces risk of cardiovascular disease.

Dosage: 2,000 IU per day; if you have vitamin D levels below 40 mg/ml, increase the dose to 10,000 IU per day and recheck labs in 6 weeks.

## Vitamin E

This vitamin is fat-soluble, which means that any excess is stored in the body. Vitamin E can be found in nuts, seeds, oils, and avocados.

Vitamin E protects nerve cells from damage due to hyperglycemia. It is an antioxidant, anti-inflammatory, and anticoagulant and reduces LDL (low quality) cholesterol. Working in tandem with the B vitamins, vitamin E helps keeps the pancreas healthy and helps prevent nerve damage. It also helps prevent kidney damage, blindness, and heart attacks. (Agur and Dalley II 2005) (Moore and Dalley 2006) Working with vitamin C, it helps keep blood vessels healthy. (Grossman 1995) (DeFronzo 2009)

Dosage: 500 IU per day.

## Vitamin B3 (Niacin)

Niacin helps to raise HDL (high quality) cholesterol, reduce LDL (low quality) cholesterol, and reduce triglycerides. Niacin protects beta islet cells from oxidative damage.

Dosage: 1500 mg per day.

### Vitamin B6
With folic acid and B12, B6 helps prevent heart attacks and nerve damage. It also helps prevent diabetic blindness and vision loss.

Dosage: 25mg per day.

### Folic Acid
This substance is needed in order for proper DNA synthesis to occur. It is anticarcinogenic and aids cell division to prevent disorders such as neural tube defects in the developing embryo. Along with B12, folic acid helps prevents strokes and loss of limbs due to diabetic complications.

Dosage: 400mcg per day.

### Vitamin B12
Vitamin B12 helps relieve depression, fatigue, and peripheral neuropathic pain. Miso has been found to be a vegan source for B12.

Dosage: 1000 mcg per day.

### Biotin
Biotin is important for diabetics because it helps to decrease insulin resistance.

Dosage: 10 mg per day.

### Magnesium
This element is involved in over 300 metabolic reactions and works best with vitamin B6. It helps to relax muscles and prevent cramping. Along with B6, it also helps relieve neuropathic pain and decrease insulin resistance.

Dosage: 500 mg per day.

### Zinc
This element is necessary for sexual maturation and reproduction. It aids in burn and wound repair, improves our ability to taste and smell,

and boosts the immune system. It also helps blood sugar get into the cells and therefore makes insulin more effective.

Dosage: 30 mg per day.

## Selenium
Selenium helps to detoxify the body and is particularly helpful in getting rid of heavy metals. It is called an insulin mimic because it helps take blood sugar into the cells. Selenium also protects against blood vessel and nerve damage from elevated blood sugars.

Dosage: 300 mcg per day.

## Potassium
Potassium is necessary for nerve transmission and skeletal muscle contraction. It strengthens bones and helps maintain acid-base balance in the body. Avocado has higher amounts of potassium than bananas.

Dosage: 5 g per day.

## Calcium
Calcium is another mineral that is essential for nerve transmission and muscle contraction. It strengthens bones and helps to increase weight loss.

Dosage: 1500 mg per day.

## Copper
Copper helps protect the insulin-producing cells in the pancreas healthy, helps prevent diabetes-related damage to blood vessels and nerves, and lowers blood sugar levels.

Dosage: 2 mg per day.

## Manganese
Manganese helps prevent damage to blood vessels and nerves.

Dosage: 4 mg per day.

### The Raw Truth: The Recipe for Reversing Diabetes

## Chromium
Chromium helps to lower LDL, total cholesterol, and triglycerides. It also helps decrease insulin resistance.

Dosage: 200 mcg per day.

## Gymnema sylvestre leaf extract
Gymnema sylvestre is a natural plant extract that helps balance blood sugars and may improve weight loss.

Dosage: 400 mg 2 times per day.

## Bitter Melon Whole Fruit Extract
This plant extract helps pathways in the diabetic liver work more efficiently and lowers blood sugar levels.

Dosage: 500 mg 2 times per day.

## Fenugreek Seed Extract
Fenugreek helps lower blood sugars and helps our liver and kidneys metabolize blood sugars more efficiently.

Dosage: 15 g per day.

## Bilberry Extract
Bilberry has been found to prevent and reduce the severity of diabetic cataracts.

Dosage: 80 mg 3 times per day.

## Mixed Bioflavonoids
Rutin and Quercitin help protect vitamins C. and E from diabetic damage. Like bilberry, bioflavonoids help keep diabetics' vision clear and sharp.

Dosage: 500 mg per day.

## Coenzyme Q10
Coenzyme Q10 helps to improve blood pressure and glycemic control.

Dosage: 200 mg per day.

## Alpha Lipoic Acid
This substance neutralizes harmful free radicals and is both a water and fat-soluble antioxidant. It helps to treat peripheral neuropathy and protects the brain and body from free radical damage that leads to aging.

Dosage: 600 mg per day.

## Digestive Enzymes
Enzymes are an essential part of the body's natural digestive process. They provide a highly concentrated form of enzymes that are naturally secreted by the pancreas and essential to the digestion of food and absorption of nutrients. The formula you choose should contain lipase, which digests fat; proteases, which digest protein; and amylases, which digest starch. Pancreatic enzyme formula provides natural nutritional support for proper digestive function.

Dosage: 2 caps with each meal.

## Probiotics
Probiotics support intestinal epithelial integrity, healthy immune response, and inflammatory balance. They promote healthy intestinal ecology to support gastrointestinal and immune health. The probiotic you take should include these five strains: Lactobacillus acidophilus, Lactobacillus rhamnosus, Lactobacillus plantarum, Bifidobacterium longum and Bifidobacterium lactis.

Dosage: 50 billion CFU per day.

# CHAPTER 13

# Plan of Action for Exercise

It is no secret that exercise, along with a raw foods diet, is a key factor in maintaining health and reversing diabetes. Moving toward a more physically active life is generally inexpensive, convenient, and easy. and it usually produces great rewards in terms of blood glucose control and a general feeling of well-being.

The benefits of exercise are well documented, and ongoing research continues to prove that it's an important activity for Americans to be engaged in. Long ago, in hunter-gatherer societies, humans' muscles got a daily workout by building shelter, running after and from animals, farming, and all the other manual chores necessary for survival. Today, however, through the use of so-called labor-saving devices, we have created an artificial environment that fosters inactivity and laziness to the extent that our muscles rarely need to be pushed very hard.

We are physically under-challenged in our day-to-day lives; this is why we admire athletes and Olympians as superior beings, even when our bodies are designed to be just as strong. We don't rake leaves or cut grass or shovel snow by hand; we don't climb stairs or even walk in airports; instead, we use elevators, escalators, and walkalators. We don't wash our clothes or our dishes or even push a vacuum by hand, and we spend more and more time watching TV, Facebooking, and Twittering than we do outdoors playing basketball, touch football, baseball, tennis, hiking, or any other recreational activities. Research shows that physical inactivity is the second leading preventable cause of death in the United States, and it's literally killing us. Stop admiring someone else's strength and regain yours.

Initially, your goal will be to work up to a routine that includes a morning and an evening workout session until your blood glucose levels are normal. Afterwards, you can reduce your routine to once per day.

**Plan of Action for Exercise**

Exercising in the morning will kick-start your metabolism, which will help you to burn more calories throughout the day. You will also receive the psychological benefits of feeling accomplished and successful about reversing your diabetes and restoring health. When you start your day with exercise and doing something good and healthy for yourself, you'll want to maintain that sense of joy, so you will continue to make healthy choices throughout the day. Exercise increases blood flow throughout the body, which also helps to stimulate the immune system and transports nutrients to all areas of the body. You will notice over time that mental fatigue and fogginess will decrease.

The main goal of exercising at night is to help you to lower your glucose levels naturally before going to bed. Typically, diabetics take medication at night to lower blood sugar levels so that they are normal in the morning. Exercise will allow your body to regain control of blood sugar regulation without having to rely on medications. Over time you will notice your fasting glucose levels returning to normal.

Exercise also benefits diabetics by giving your beta cells a break from excessive insulin production. Whenever you actively use a muscle, you burn both fatty acids and glucose. During and after periods of activity, the beta cells in your pancreas sense your falling glucose level, so they relax their output of insulin. At first you may notice an increase in your glucose levels following exercise, but this will regulate over time.

These lower insulin levels also signal your liver to empty its glucose reserves (glycogen) into the blood to supply the muscles with needed energy. As physical activity continues, the liver converts amino acids, lactic acid, and fats into glucose to supply the muscles. If the activity continues long enough, even the body's fat cells get into the game. They compensate for the reduced fatty acid levels in your blood by converting their stored triglycerides into fatty acids.

Fortunately, exercise is not an all or nothing endeavor. A little is better than none and you can do something today, so don't worry about what you will do next month. This perspective is hard for anyone who expects a lot from themselves and sets long-term fitness goals. Don't expect results overnight. But do expect to take small steps every day.

Your exercise program doesn't need to be elaborate. But it does require you to sweat. You should break a sweat during each workout.

Sometimes exercise requires motivation, so getting together with a friend to exercise is a great plan. Surround yourself with people who are healthy and active. Odds are it will be easier for you to stay active as well. Check in with your doctor to get help in setting attainable, yet realistic goals. Try to set a plan to go faster, farther, or longer with your routine.

Try a variety of exercises to see which type works best for you. Some people prefer running on a treadmill, while others prefer running on a track. You may need to try a variety of activities before you find one that you really like and want to do long term. Sign up for a yoga class or Pilates. Try running or biking instead of walking, go with others or go alone, or try exercising at different times of the day. Keep your options open and find exercises you enjoy. Exercise is not meant to be a chore; rather, it should be a part of your daily routine.

In the beginning, you can create an exercise log book. Simply writing down what you did, how long you did it, and how you felt can be a great motivator. Not only can you view your progress and look back at your accomplishments, but you can plan ahead and decide where you want to be in a week, a month, or in the long term. You can also use this log to review your workout plan with your doctor.

The key to a successful workout plan is to put it at the top of your priorities list. If your exercise plans and goals are at the bottom, you will never reach them. You have to believe that getting healthy is important enough for you to make it happen. Take a serious look at your words, desires, and behavior. Now is the time to take back control of your health and break the vicious cycle of helplessness. Get honest with yourself about what you really want and how much you are willing to work to make it happen. You'll see how easily it falls into place once you put your energy into taking action rather than making excuses.

## Stretching

One of the biggest mistakes people make when exercising isn't something they do, but something they don't do. You may think that stretching your hamstrings and calves is just something to be done if you have a few extra minutes before or after pounding out some miles on the treadmill, and your main concern is getting the workout done right.

Well, not so fast! Stretching may help you improve flexibility, and better flexibility may improve your performance in physical activities or decrease your risk of injury by helping your joints move through their full range of motion.

If you have short, tight muscles and are not as limber as others, you will have your work cut out for you. However, people in this group need to stretch consistently in order to prevent the physiological loss of flexibility that comes with age, and their tight muscles feel much better after moderate stretching.

Reduced muscle tension that results from stretching improves the range of joint movement and muscle coordination, and it increases blood circulation to produce higher energy levels. The more frequently you stretch, the more quickly you will gain flexibility, though big changes take time. After every exercise session, try to stretch your arms, your back from the base of your neck to the top of your sacrum (the lowest part of your back), and your legs from toes to hips. Stretch at least three or four times a week. Do each stretch to the point of "mild discomfort" and hold each stretch for 10-30 seconds.

If you have long, thin muscles, you tend to be more limber and flexible. Generally, maintaining appropriate flexibility and range of joint motion is good for people of any muscle type. However, those who fall into this category need to be extra vigilant. Over-stretching can cause muscle and/or tendon strain, most commonly in the neck, shoulder, hips, legs, and back. Less commonly, partial disclocation or complete dislocation of joints can occur. For those who are extremely flexible, over-stretching is a huge temptation. You sometimes may want to push beyond what you can safely do. You will have to use reason and common sense. If you feel pain, damage may already have been done.

The rules of stretching are basic. If it hurts, you've gone too far. Everyone who stretches should be careful not to stretch to the point of even moderate pain. Be careful not to stretch a muscle beyond its natural range, which you can see and feel. Breathe while stretching, so as not to deprive your muscles of the oxygen they need.

Before you plunge into stretching, make sure you do it safely and effectively. While you can stretch anytime, anywhere (in your home, at the office, in an airport, or at the gym), you want to be sure to use proper technique. Stretching incorrectly can actually do more harm than good. Here are some tips for correct and safe stretching.

- Don't consider stretching a warm-up. You may hurt yourself if you stretch cold muscles. So, before stretching, warm up with light walking, jogging, or biking at low intensity for five to ten minutes. Or better yet, stretch after you exercise when your muscles are warmed up. Also, consider holding off on stretching before an intense activity, such as sprinting or track and field activities. Some research suggests that pre-event stretching before these types of events may actually decrease performance.

- Focus on major muscle groups. When you're stretching, focus on your calves, thighs, hips, lower back, neck, and shoulders. Also stretch muscles and joints that you routinely use at work or play. And make sure that you stretch both sides. For instance, if you stretch your left hamstring, be sure to stretch your right hamstring, too.

- Don't bounce. Bouncing as you stretch can cause small tears in the muscle. These tears leave scar tissue as the muscle heals, which tightens the muscle even further, making you less flexible and more prone to pain. So, hold each stretch for about 30 seconds. Repeat each stretch three or four times.

- Don't aim for pain. Expect to feel tension while you're stretching, but not pain. If it hurts, you've pushed too far. Back off to the point where you don't feel any pain, then hold the stretch.

- Some evidence suggests that it's helpful to do stretches that area tailored for your sport or activity. If you play soccer, for instance, you're more vulnerable to hamstring strains, so you would want to opt for stretches that help your hamstrings. Make your stretches sport specific.

- Keep up with your stretching. Stretching can be time-consuming. But you can achieve the best benefits by stretching regularly, at least two to three times per week. If you don't stretch regularly, you risk losing any benefits that stretching offered. For instance, if stretching helped you increase your range of motion, and you stop stretching, your range of motion may decrease again.

- Bring movement into your stretching. Gentle movement can help you be more flexible in specific movements. The gentle movements of tai chi, for instance, may be a good way to stretch. And if you're going to perform a specific activity, such as a front kick in martial arts, do the move slowly and at low intensity at first to get your muscles used to it. Then speed up gradually as your muscles become accustomed to the motion.

- Know when to exercise caution. In some cases, especially if you have a chronic condition or injury, you may need to be careful while stretching and make sure your stretching routine does not aggravate the problem. For example, if you already have a strained muscle, stretching it may cause further harm.

- Don't fall into the error of thinking that because you stretch you can't get injured. For instance, stretching won't prevent an overuse injury. If you have any health concerns, talk to your doctor or physical therapist about the best way to stretch.

## Types of Exercise

### Aerobic
Cardiovascular exercise is also known as aerobic (uses oxygen) exercise;

it helps to make your heart and lungs stronger. Walking, jogging, running, swimming, elliptical cross-training, biking, using a Stairmaster, and rowing are common forms of aerobic exercise. Cardiovascular health benefits include lowering blood pressure, burning lots of calories, reduced risk of heart disease, improved blood cholesterol and triglyceride levels, improved heart function, reduced risk of osteoporosis, and improved muscle mass.

In order to reverse your diabetes it is important to engage in aerobic exercise several times per week. You should work your way up to 20 to 60 minutes of moderate to intense physical activity five to seven days per week. Working up to this level is important because this is the only way to get into the zone that challenges your heart and lungs. In order to do this, it's necessary to sustain your workout for 20 minutes or more at least three times per week.

You can calculate your target heart rate by using this formula:

$$220 - \text{your age} \times 70\%$$

For example: 220-40 years = 180 x 0.7= 126. In that example, the ideal workout zone is a heart rate of 126 beats per minute. If your heart rate halfway through your workout is over that 70% mark, you can reduce your intensity a little. If you are under the 70% mark, however, then you need to pick up the pace.

You can calculate your heart rate by checking you pulse for 6 seconds and adding a zero at the end (i.e. 8 beats in 6 seconds will equal a heart rate of 80 beats per minute). Another way to calculate your heart rate is to get a pulse monitor or use the monitor on the aerobic equipment at the gym.

Running is one of the best options for burning calories and regulating your blood sugar levels. In addition, it strengthens your heart, lungs, and legs. Running has the same effects on the body whether it's done outside or on a treadmill.

Once you begin an exercise session, it will take your body around 20 minutes to get warmed up. Your warm-up time will decrease as your fitness level increases. If you have bad knees, using an elliptical machine or swimming are great alternatives to running.

## Anaerobic

The term "anaerobic" means "without oxygen." Anaerobic exercises are those that do not use oxygen for energy. It's impossible to do anaerobic exercise for a long period of time because the lack of oxygen results in a by-product called lactic acid in the muscles.

It is inefficient for the body to use muscles without oxygen at a high intensity for a short period of time because the buildup of lactic acid affects muscle action and function and can contribute to muscle fatigue. The body has to convert lactic acid to pyruvate or glucose during a recovery period before another anaerobic exercise can be performed. This is why you have to include recovery periods while doing anaerobic exercise. During the recovery period, the muscles will use oxygen to assist in replenishing the energy that was used during the anaerobic exercise.

Compared with aerobic exercise, anaerobic exercise requires a person to move at an increased pace or to perform the exercise with greater effort. In theory, exercising anaerobically can cause the body to burn more calories than aerobic exercising. However, during anaerobic exercise, oxygen is not delivered in sufficient quantities to allow the cells to continue burning fat. Instead, the muscle cells burn mainly carbohydrates, which burn more quickly and do not require oxygen. Common examples of anaerobic exercise include sprinting, push-ups, pull-ups, and lifting weights. It is usually recommended that you do anaerobic exercises for 10 to 20 minutes two to three times a week in addition to aerobic exercise.

Anaerobic exercises involve repetition. Beginning exercisers may want to start with one set of 10 to 15 repetitions and build up to two or three sets as your muscles become stronger. If you are using weights, choose one that is about half of what would require your maximum effort to lift for one repetition. It is important to focus on slow rhythmic breathing and to try to avoid holding your breath, since holding your breath or straining during exercise can promote injury.

**The Raw Truth: The Recipe for Reversing Diabetes**

Anaerobic exercise is not nearly as effective for directly burning fat as aerobic exercise is. However, anaerobic exercise helps burn fat indirectly by increasing the metabolic rate after the exercise session. Because anaerobic exercise builds muscle and muscle requires energy in the form of calories, you'll burn more calories even when your body is at rest. Other health benefits from anaerobic exercise include an overall increased metabolism, the ability to consume more calories without gaining weight due to the higher metabolism, the development of lean muscle mass, and the toning and firming of muscles.

Resistance training is any exercise that causes the muscles to contract against an external resistance, conducted with the expectation of increasing strength, tone, mass, and/or endurance. The external resistance can be dumbbells, rubber exercise tubing, your own body weight, bricks, bottles of water, or any other object that causes the muscles to contract.

Resistance training works by causing microscopic damage or tears to the muscle cells, which the body will then quickly repair to help the muscles regenerate and grow stronger. The breakdown of the muscle fiber is called "catabolism," and the repair and re-growth of the muscle tissue is called "anabolism." This may sound strange, but many biological processes of growth in the body require some breakdown prior to re-growth. For instance, bones must be broken down (catabolism) before calcium and other growth factors repair the bone and make it stronger (anabolism). After a resistance training session, testosterone, insulin-like growth factor, growth hormone, protein, and other nutrients rush to the muscle to help repair it and make it stronger. Your muscles heal and grow when you aren't working out, so that's why it's important to leave time between workouts for recovery.

If you are a beginner or someone who is just starting to exercise again after years of a more sedentary lifestyle, then start small. Start with one set of 8 to 10 different exercises for the major muscle groups, and do 10 to 15 repetitions of each, two to three days per week. As your strength improves, increase the amount of sets you perform for each exercise. For those of you that are older or in far less then optimal shape, 8-12 repetitions may be more appropriate.

Your exercise routine will work off of the principles of progressive overload. Progressive overload is a simple concept to understand. When you first start to lift a weight, it may be too heavy to lift more then a few times. As your muscles grow, however, it becomes easier and easier to lift the same amount of weight. When lifting that weight 12-15 times becomes easy, you will then increase the weight and lift that new weight until you can once again do 12-15 repetitions with ease. Typically every time you add new weight, you lift fewer reps, but then, as your muscles grow stronger, you perform more reps. The principle of progressive overload is universally accepted as the model that creates the greatest gains in strength.

One of the best pieces of equipment you can use during your resistance training is your own body. Push-ups, pull-ups, dips, sit-ups, squats, lunges, and step-ups are just some of the exercises that you can do to strengthen your body. The advantage of these exercises is that you can do most of them anywhere.

Pull-ups strengthen the arms, back, and shoulders. Some people can't do even a single pull-up. What you can do to help is stand on a chair under a pull-up bar to lighten the load as you pull up (the chair supports some of your body weight). Outdoors you can do pull-ups on a tree limb and ask a friend to support some of your weight by holding your feet!

Push-ups strengthen the arms, chest, and shoulders. Don't worry if you can't do a traditional push-up. Here's a sequence that will get you there: start with the wall push-up. Just like it sounds, lean against a wall about two feet from the wall with your back straight and push back and forth. When wall push-ups are easy, lean against a countertop. When leaning against the counter gets easy, get on the floor on your knees and push against the edge of a sofa or your bed. When the sofa gets easy, do a knee push-up on the floor. Like it sounds, you are on your knees with your back straight and you lower yourself to the floor and then back up again. Most people find that once they can do 20-25 knee push-ups on the floor, they can do one regular push-up (with knees off the floor).

No one method of resistance exercise is superior to the other. As long as your muscles are contracting against external resistance — whether it's dumbbells, machines, tubing, your own body weight, bottles of water, or cinder blocks — the exercises will work to build your body's strength and tone.

Assess your skills. Consider hiring a fitness trainer to work with you at a gym or at your home if you're a beginner. It's difficult to learn how to lift weights on your own, equipped with just a book or even a video. You can do it, but the hands-on approach with a trainer is superior. You don't need to use the trainer forever, either. You can start by having the trainer design a plan for you and show you how to do it. Then, depending on your skill, you might only need a couple of sessions and then a periodic follow-up with the trainer, say, once every one to two months. Learning how to lift weights properly will give you the confidence you need to lift on your own and get stronger and stronger.

You goal may be to lose weight, tone up, and get stronger. The good news is that any lifting will tone you up and give you strength. Fat loss is mostly achieved via aerobic exercise. You can expect strength gains in just a few weeks. Tone comes later, and how much muscle you see depends on how much excess body fat you have. For instance, if you have lots of excess fat on the back of your arms, then you won't see the triceps muscles right away; likewise, if you have excess fat on your belly, then you won't see six-pack abs until you reduce or eliminate the fat.

## Design Your Plan

### Weights

Beginners should start with weights that can be lifted 10-12 reps to fatigue with good form. Fatigue means that you cannot lift the weight one more time with good form. If you have to lean back or throw the weight up, then it's too heavy. Lifting 10-12 reps to fatigue will maximize your strength gains and minimize the risk of overtraining or injury.

# Plan of Action for Exercise

## Sets
Beginners can start with one set per exercise. You can do more if you have time, but research shows that one set for beginners is enough to yield significant gains in strength.

## Time Between Sets
Rest less than one minute between sets if you want to develop endurance and tone. Rest up to three minutes if you want to focus more on strength; the extra recovery time allows the muscles to work harder and lift more on the next set.

## Order of Exercises
Design your plan so that large muscle groups are worked before smaller groups. The theory is that if you fatigue a smaller muscle group first, then the larger group won't work as hard as it can. For example, work the chest or back before shoulders, biceps or triceps; shoulders before biceps or triceps; and quads or hamstrings before calves or abs.

Compound exercises should come before isolation exercises. For example, do the bench press before dumbbell flies; overhead press before lateral raises; squats before leg extensions; and Romanian deadlifts before leg curls.

Finally, free weight/body weight exercises should come before using exercise machines. For example, do squats or deadlifts before leg presses; barbell bench press before incline machine press; and pull-ups before chest supported machine rows.

This is the ideal way to work out, but remember that right now the most important thing for you to do is simply to work out.

## Exercises
Select one to two exercises per muscle group. Here's a list of at least two exercises for each group using dumbbells and machines in an order of larger to smaller muscle groups. All of these exercises and the order of exercises are suitable for beginners

## Upper body workout
Chest: dumbbell press, dumbbell flies, chest press, cable flies (crossovers); or

Back: bent-over-row, cable row, pull-down.

Followed by shoulders: side lateral raise, front raise, upright row.

Arms: biceps curls, triceps kickbacks, triceps press-downs on pull-down machine.

## Lower body workout
Legs: squats, leg extensions, and curls on the machines, leg press on the machine.

Followed by abs: crunches, knee-drop crunches for the oblique muscles on the side of the abdomen (drop the knees to one side and crunch up).

## Rest and recovery
Remember that muscles grow during downtime, not when you train, so allow a day or two between workouts when you first get started so that the muscles can recover and grow. You should show up at your workouts refreshed and at least as strong as the previous workout. (There will be days when you don't feel stronger than the previous day, and you should expect them. Don't get discouraged when this happens.)

## Splits
"Split" is a term used to describe how you organize your workout. For instance, you might decide to work only your chest on day one and your back on day two. This is the type of lifting you do once you get stronger and more experienced. This is not necessary or recommended for beginners because it's too intense. It's not only unnecessary, but it could lead to injury or overtraining (burnout).

Below is a three-day per week beginner program broken up by muscle group.

**Day one:** chest (bench press with bar or dumbbell press, flies, push-ups), triceps (bench dips, kickbacks), legs (squats or leg press, leg extension, leg curl)

**Day two:** back (bent-over rows or seated cable rows), biceps (curls, standing or seated)

**Day three:** shoulders (lateral raises, front raises), legs (squats or leg press, leg extension, leg curl)

Work the abs at each workout. Crunches are a good way to start, and below are some excellent advanced abdominal exercises. Make sure to stretch your lower back before and after doing them.

## Bicycle maneuver

Lie flat on the floor with your lower back pressed to the ground. Put your hands beside your head. Bring your knees up to about a 45-degree angle and slowly go through a bicycle pedal motion. Touch your left elbow to your right knee, then your right elbow to your left knee. Keep even, relaxed breathing throughout.

## Captain's chair

Stabilize your upper body by gripping the hand holds and lightly pressing your lower back against the back pad. The starting position begins with you holding your body up with legs dangling below. Now slowly lift your knees in toward your chest. The motion should be controlled and deliberate as you bring the knees up and return them back to the starting position.

## Crunch on exercise ball

Sit on the ball with your feet flat on the floor. Let the ball roll back slowly. Now lie back on the ball until your thighs and torso are parallel with the floor. Cross your arms over your chest and slightly tuck your chin in toward your chest. Contract your abdominals, raising your torso to no more than 45 degrees. For better balance, spread your feet wider apart. To challenge the obliques, make the exercise less stable by moving your feet closer together. Exhale as you contract; inhale as you return to the starting position.

## Vertical leg crunch

Lie flat on the floor with your lower back pressed to the ground. Put your hands behind your head for support. Extend your legs straight up in the air, crossed at the ankles with a slight bend in the knee. Contract your abdominal muscles by lifting your torso toward your knees. Make sure to keep your chin off your chest with each contraction. Exhale as you contract upward, and inhale as you return to the starting position.

## Reverse crunch

Lie flat on the floor with your lower back pressed to the ground. Put your hands beside your head or extend them out flat to your sides — whatever feels most comfortable. Crossing your feet at the ankles, lift your feet off the ground to the point where your knees create a 90-degree angle. Once in this position, press your lower back on the floor as you contract your abdominal muscles. Your hips will slightly rotate, and your legs will reach toward the ceiling with each contraction. Exhale as you contract, and inhale as you return to the starting position.

Be sure to not overdo your workout. If you have type 1 diabetes and are in ketoacidosis, avoid exercise because it can worsen hyperglycemia and ketosis. However, if you simply have hyperglycemia, you feel well, and you are negative for ketones in your blood and/or urine, then it is not necessary for you to postpone exercising.

# CHAPTER 14

# Living Raw for Life

Diabetes is the only disease where you can see in real time how your actions affect your state of health: what you eat starts affecting your blood sugar levels in a matter of minutes. The foods you are eating have to remain in your consciousness, and you have to remember, "you are what you eat." If you eat foods that are full of life and nutrients, then your body and health will benefit. If you eat foods that are full of dead flesh and low in nutrients, then your body and health will suffer.

The recipe for health has already been designed for you by nature and it is in the foods that we eat. The main ingredients in the recipe for health are raw foods, exercise, and the knowledge that you are responsible for your health.

Raw food veganism is a vegan lifestyle that consists of unprocessed, raw plant foods that have not been heated to temperatures above approximately 118 degrees Fahrenheit. Typical foods on this raw vegan diet include fruit, vegetables, nuts, seeds, and sprouted grains and legumes. During this time of your healing phase, fruits are to be avoided.

Eating foods in their raw, uncooked state gives you all the nutrients your body needs for life. Raw foods provide enzymes that help our body digest the foods we are eating. When we cook foods at temperatures above 180 degrees for prolonged times, those enzymes are destroyed and denatured to a configuration that is not normal for the body. Enzymes denatured by stomach acid are simply deactivated and become active again after leaving the acidic environment. When we consume cooked foods, the enzymes that are lost during the cooking process have to be generated by the body. This creates extra work and leads to aging.

**The Raw Truth: The Recipe for Reversing Diabetes**

Nearly every food preparation process reduces the amount of nutrients in food. In particular, processes that expose foods to high levels of heat, light, and/or oxygen cause the greatest nutrient loss. These nutrients are essential for the body to function at its most efficiently while doing everything from building tissue to activating key enzymes. Commercially grown foods may already be low in nutrients due to the decreased time allowed for vegetables to grow before they are harvested. Cooking these foods just further depletes the nutrients.

By now you should know that raw plant foods do provide adequate protein. The truth is that 20-50% of calories in vegetables come from protein. Sprouted seeds, beans, and grains contain 10-15% protein. Fruits have about 5% of their calories from protein. So if a rawfoodist ate 2000 calories that were made up of 10% protein, that would be 200 calories or 50 g of protein. (There are 4 calories in 1 g of protein.) As you can see, this person would still be getting enough protein in their diet.

The biggest benefit of a raw food diet, however, is that the food is still alive and retains its electromagnetic energy that resonates throughout your body while you eat it. It is rebalancing you and connecting you with the source of life. Eating raw foods is the equivalent of recharging your life battery, providing you with the energy to continue living. After the detox phase, you will notice that your energy, mood, and attitude will improve. Be full of life!

Foods to eat are listed below in the phase system chart. For diabetes and other major illnesses, start off in phase 1 for a minimum of thirty days. It may take longer to reverse diabetes. The goal is to have your blood sugar levels stable for three weeks before adding in higher glycemic foods from the other phases.

Phase 1 foods are low on the glycemic index and promote healing. These foods act like a roto-rooter that cleans out your blood vessels, removing bad fat and cholesterol and replacing them with good fat and cholesterol. Once your health is fully restored, you can incorporate foods from phase 2 and minimal use phase 2 categories. You will see that you have a wide variety of foods to eat.

- **Phase 1**: Used for detoxification and reversal of major disease
- **Phase 1.5**: Used after detoxification or for moderate disease
- **Phase 2**: Used for maintenance of health after reversing disease or to remain healthy
- **Phase 2 Minimal use**: Eat foods in this group occasionally
- **Foods to avoid**: Foods in this group should not be consumed due to their inflammatory and disease promoting nature

## Phase 1

- nuts and seeds
- all greens
- all vegetables (except those listed elsewhere)
- sea vegetables
- coconut pulp
- tomatoes
- avocadoes
- cucumber
- red bell pepper
- carrots (raw)
- summer squash (raw): yellow squash, patti pan
- flax oil
- hemp oil
- extra virgin olive oil
- sesame oil
- almond oil
- sunflower oil
- coconut oil (butter)
- lemons
- limes
- Klamath lake algae
- super green powders
- mushrooms (raw)
- Bragg Liquid Aminos
- miso
- apple cider vinegar
- yacon syrup
- stevia

**The Raw Truth: The Recipe for Reversing Diabetes**

## Phase 1.5
- hard squash (raw)
- coconut water (diluted with other ingredients)
- grapefruit
- raspberries
strawberries
cherries
- blueberries
- goji berries
- cranberries (fresh, unsweetened)
- non stored grains:
  - wild rice
  - quinoa
  - millet
  - buckwheat
  - spelt
  - amaranth
- fermented foods:
  - sauerkraut
  - kefir

## Phase 2
- sweet potatoes (raw)
- yams (raw)
- pumpkin (raw)
- parsnips (raw)
- rutabaga (raw)
- beets (raw)
- oranges
- pears
- apples
- plums
- peaches
- pomegranates
- blackberries
- grapefruit juice (diluted with water)
- carob (raw)
- bee pollen
- unfermented soy products

## Phase 2 Minimal use
- sweet potatoes (cooked)
- rutabaga (cooked)
- beets (cooked)
- hard squash (cooked)
- summer squash (cooked)
- carrot juice
- orange juice
- apricots
- grapes
- figs
- raisins
- melons
- bananas
- mangos

- papaya
- kiwi
- pineapple
- sapote
- cherimoya
- rambutian
- durian
- dates

- cashews
- dried fruits
- fresh, raw fruit juices
- seed cheese
- mushrooms (cooked)
- cooked, organic whole foods
- Nama Shoyu

## Foods to Avoid
- all animal products:
- flesh
- eggs
- dairy
- all processed foods
- all grains (except those listed)
- corn
- white potatoes
- white flour
- white rice
- honey
- alcohol

- sugar
- coffee
- tobacco
- heated oils (except coconut oil)
- peanuts
- brewer's yeast
- nutritional yeast
- cottonseed
- yeast
- bottled juices

## Juicing

Juicing is a fun way to get the whole family involved in nutrition. Kids often do not like to eat their green vegetables because they were introduced at such a young age, as early as when they were in the womb, to the processed foods available in our modern world. Juicing helps to restore taste and nutrition.

Juicing extracts the juice from fresh fruits or vegetables. The result is a liquid that contains most of the vitamins, minerals, and phytonutrients found in the whole fruit. However, whole fruits and vegetables also have healthy fiber, which is lost during most juicing. Because of the loss of fiber, people with type 2 diabetes should initially avoid juicing. Juicing is more beneficial for people with type 1 diabetes.

Juices should be prepared fresh daily and consumed within 24 hours. Juice is full of nutrients that can be used as food by harmful bacteria. To avoid contamination, put the leftover juice in a sealed glass and refrigerate. When juicing, try to keep some of the pulp, which can later be used in recipes for breads and crackers.

Consuming freshly juiced organic vegetables provides you with a lot of nutrients. Those nutrients are quickly absorbed by the body and require less digesting. You get all these minerals and nutrients, with very few calories, from juice. Juicing allows you to mix and match different types of vegetables to create delicious juices that will be enjoyed by everyone.

## Water

Water is vital to the survival of the human body. The body cannot work without it, just as a car cannot run without gas and oil. In fact, all the cell and organ functions that make up our entire anatomy and physiology depend on water.

Water makes up more than two-thirds of a human's body weight, and without water, we would die in a few days. The human brain is made up of 95% water, blood is 82% water, and the lungs 90% water. A mere 2% drop in our body's water supply can trigger signs of dehydration: fuzzy short-term memory, trouble with basic math, and difficulty focusing on smaller print.

Dehydration can often be interpreted as hunger. Before reaching for food, drink water and see how you feel afterwards. It really could be all your body needed. You can even boost the benefits of your water by adding an electrolyte mix to it.

Your goal is to drink half of your body weight in ounces of purified water (i.e. a 120-pound person should drink at least 60 ounces of water daily). Add an additional eight ounces of water if you are pregnant.

Water is far from inanimate; it is actually alive and responsive to our every thought and emotion. Be conscious of this when consuming water and channel your thoughts to be healing and loving; those vibratory energies will be carried throughout your body as the water nourishes and cleanses it.

## Sprouting and Soaking

Soaking and sprouting nuts, seeds, and grains make them more bioactive. These benefits include increased enzyme activity and removal of tannins and phytic acid, which leads to increased digestibility and greater absorption of the food's nutrients by the body. When soaked, nuts and seeds will begin the sprouting process, which bumps up their nutrient profiles considerably.

| Seed, Nut or Grain | Soak Time (Hours) | Sprout Time (Days) |
|---|---|---|
| Almonds | 8-12 | N/A |
| Barley | 6-8 | 2 |
| Buckwheat | 6 | 2 |
| Cashews | 4-6 | N/A |
| Chickpeas | 8-12 | 2-3 |
| Flax Seeds | 0.5 | 1 |
| Kamut | 7 | 2-3 |
| Lentil Beans | 7 | 3 |
| Oat Groats | 6 | 2 |
| Quinoa | 2 | 1 |
| Rye | 8 | 3 |
| Sesame Seeds | 6 | 2 |
| Spelt | 7 | 2 |
| Walnuts | 4 | N/A |
| Wheat Berries | 7 | 2-3 |
| Wild Rice | 9 | 3-5 |
| All Other nuts | 6 | N/A |

## Equipment You Need to Get Started

### Food Dehydrator

Your food dehydrator will replace your oven. This is what we use to "bake" cookies, pies, entrees, breads, crackers, snacks, and other foods. With a food dehydrator you are able to remove moisture without killing the food. The enzymes are still intact and functional at temperatures up to 118 degrees. At temperatures from 118 to about 140 degrees, many enzymes in food still function, but do so at a lower efficiency. Cooking food above 158 degrees destroys almost all the enzymes in the food. So it is best to dehydrate your food at temperatures below 118 degrees Fahrenheit in order to maintain enzyme function.

If you are not ready to purchase a dehydrator, you can use your oven at its lowest temperature setting and keep the door open. However, this will be less efficient and more costly than purchasing a dehydrator.

### Food processor

A food processor is such a help in the kitchen and cuts down on food prep time. It shreds, mixes, chops, minces, and blends. You will use this to make pate and dough for breads and crackers.

### Juicer

This appliance is useful for preparing fresh, nutritious juices. There are several types of juicers: centrifugal, masticating, and triturating.

If you have limited time in your day and want to make fresh juice as quickly as possible, then a centrifugal juice extractor is your best choice. Centrifugal juice extractors are generally the cheapest of the various kinds of electric juicers available, so they are also a great choice for a limited budget.

In comparison to centrifugal juicers, masticating juicers run at a slower speed and drastically reduce the amount of heat that fruits and vegetables are subject to. This preserves a lot more of the living enzymes and antioxidants, producing a juice that better promotes health. The juice yield, and therefore the nutritional value, is higher than that of a centrifugal juicer.

Triturating juice extractors are the elite of juice extractors. They work in the same way as a masticating juicer but have two gears instead of just one. The gears run side by side and extremely close together. As vegetables pass through the gears, they get just about every last drop of juice squeezed out of them at a very slow speed. So triturating juice extractors are a little more effective than single gear masticating juicers and produce a higher yield and less oxidation.

## Blender
Your blender will be very useful for preparing soups, sauces, smoothies, and puddings. It is the most common instrument used in preparing raw foods.

## Coffee Grinder
Coffee grinders can help you make flour from nuts and seeds and grind spices.

## Knives
A raw diet involves a lot of food preparation and chopping and cutting of vegetables. Getting used to using a kitchen knife set will save you time and energy. Talk with a cutlery expert to help you select a set that will be best for you.

# CHAPTER 15

# Pulling it All together

Get started: Review Chapter 10: Escaping the Healthcare Model and Chapter 12: Supplements

Check in with your doctor: Have your physician order the labs found in Chapter 10 and devise a plan that includes supplements found in Chapter 12. Constantly educate yourself on what it takes to be healthy and retrain your thinking and relationship with food.

Eating: Review Chapter 15: Living Raw for Life. Eat and prepare foods from phase 1 for at least three weeks after blood sugar levels have stabilized before moving on to phase 1.5 and phase 2.

**Juicing**
For type 1 diabetes: Do not start off with a juice feast. I find that it is difficult to regulate blood sugar levels by consuming mostly juice because the fiber content necessary to decrease absorption is not present. After blood sugar levels have stabilized, then you will be able to drink juices prepared from foods in phase 1. After several months of stable blood sugar levels, you may add phase 1.5 and phase 2 foods to your juices.

For types 1.5 and 2 diabetes, prediabetes, and gestational diabetes: Green juice feasting works quickly to lower blood sugar levels and will reduce fat. Some people may be able to maintain a juice feast for as long as 60 days. Use foods from phase 1 until three weeks after blood sugar levels have stabilized. Then you may add foods from phase 1.5 and phase 2.

Water: Drink 20 ounces of clean water upon waking. Every day, your water intake in ounces should correspond to half your body weight in pounds.

Exercise: Review Chapter 13: Plan of Action for Exercise. Engage in daily exercise. Your goal is to burn at least 250 calories during each workout. Engage in aerobic exercise to burn fat and lose weight. Engage in anaerobic exercise to increase muscle mass and strength.

Colonics: Review Chapter 11: Detoxification. Do a colonic at least once per week during the initial detoxification phase.

## Tracking Your Progress

Monitor your fasting and two-hour postprandial blood sugar levels to see how well your diet and exercise program is working for you.

Monitor body composition with a scale that tracks weight, body fat percentage, bone mass percentage, water percentage, and BMI. You can calculate your muscle percentage by using the following formula:

Muscle Percentage = 100% - body fat % - Water % - bone mass %

For example, if your body fat is 8%, your water content 62%, and bone mass 8.4%, your calculation would look like this:

100% - 8% body fat - 62% water - 8.4% bone = 21.6 % muscle

By keeping track of these numbers, you can tailor your workout plan to gain more muscle or burn more fat.

BMI Ranges: Underweight: <18.5; Normal weight: 18.5-24.9; Overweight: 25-29.9; Obese: ≥ 30

| Date | Weight (lbs.) | BMI | Fat% | Water% | Bone% | Muscle% | Blood sugar fasting | 2 hrs. after eating | Blood sugar before bed |
|---|---|---|---|---|---|---|---|---|---|
| 8-4 | 268 | 46 | 35 | 48 | 8.6 | 8.4 | 290 | 340 | 300 |
| 6 after | 194 | 33.3 | 25 | 55 | 8.4 | 11.6 | 94 | <146 | <100 |

You can calculate your body composition using this example:

Fat %= 35%; Weight is 268 lbs.

268 lbs x 0.35 = 93.8 lbs. of fat.

**The Raw Truth: The Recipe for Reversing Diabetes**

One pound of fat has 3500 calories of energy. One pound of muscle has 700 calories of energy. Therefore, one pound of fat has enough energy to produce 5 pounds of muscle.

Water %= 48%; Weight is 268 lbs

268lbs x 0.48 = 128.64 lbs. of water. This may sound like a lot of water, but this person is actually dehydrated. We want water percentage to be above 60%.

This person has a lot of work to do. But it can be done and has been done following the recipe laid out in this book.

# RAW FOOD RECIPES

**Dressings/Sauces/Condiments**

Ranch Dressing ..........................106
Lemon-Basil Vinaigrette ........106
Caesar Dressing ........................107
Italian Dressing ........................107
Mustard......................................107
Ginger Tahini Miso Dressing..108
Chipotle Sauce ........................108
Cheese Sauce ..............................109
Mayonnaise..................................109
Ketchup ......................................109
Cocktail Sauce ..........................110
Guacamole..................................110
Sour Cream ................................110
Sweet and Sour ........................111
BBQ Sauce ................................111
Pizza Sauce I..............................112
Peanut Sauce ............................112
Cheddar Cheese Sauce ............113
Sour Cream and Onion Dip ....113
Pad Thai Sauce..........................113
Salsa ..........................................114
Vinaigrette ................................114
 Pesto ........................................114
Lemon Vinaigrette Dressing....115
Caesar Dressing II......................115
Ricotta Cheese ..........................115
Chow Mein Sauce ....................116
Mushroom Gravy......................116

**Salads**

Kale Salad with Pine Nuts, Apricots, and Cheese Sauce..........................................117
Thai Tomato Salad....................117
Green House Salad ..................118
Taco Salad..................................118
Caesar Salad..............................118
Spinach Salad with Red Onion and Hazelnuts ........................119
Farmer's Salad ..........................119
Tomato-Radicchio with Basil Vinaigrette..............................120
Candied Walnut Salad ............120
Curry Cabbage Salad ..............121
Pad Thai Salad ..........................121
Cole Slaw..................................122
Italian Pesto Salad ..................122
Tomato Basil Salad ..................123
Broccoli Salad............................123
Cherry Tomato Cucumber Salad......................................124
Carrot Salad ..............................124
Cucumber Salad........................125
Jicama Salad ............................125
Seaweed and Kale Salad1........126
Make It Work Salad ................126

**Breakfast**

Pecan Porridge ..........................127

Pecan and Blueberry Porridge .................................. 127
Macadamia Nut Porridge ........ 127
Granola ........................................... 128
Buckwheat Granola ................... 128
Living Bagel ................................. 129

**Entrees**
Pizza Crust .................................... 130
Cheeze ........................................... 131
Pizza Sauce II .............................. 131
Taco ................................................ 132
Spring Rolls ................................. 132
Massaman ..................................... 133
Tempura Vegetables ................. 134
Life Burgers ................................. 134
Living Life Eggplant "Bacon" Burgers ..................................... 135
Chesapeake Bay Nori Rolls .... 136
Lasagna .......................................... 138
Pasta Marinara or Pesto .......... 138
Chow Mein .................................... 139
Chipotle Lime Tacos ................. 139
Tuna Salad .................................... 140
Sloppy Joe .................................... 140
Chicken Salad ............................. 141
Crab Cakes ................................... 141
Eggplant Bacon .......................... 142
Veggie Fajitas .............................. 143
Spinach Lasagna ........................ 144
Stuffed Bell Peppers ................. 145

**Snacks/Appetizers**
Red Bell Pepper Hummus ...... 146
Hummus ........................................ 146
Egg-less Salad ............................ 147
Mashed Potatoes ...................... 147
"Rice" ............................................. 148
Zucchini Fries ............................. 148
Tomato Chips ............................. 149

**Juices/Smoothies/Milks**
Blood Orange Christian .......... 150
Banana Breakfast Shake .......... 150
Almond & Banana Smoothie 150
Pineapple Melon Smoothie .... 151
Orange and Red Kicker ........... 151
Bitter Sweet Beet Smoothie .. 151
Tropical Strawberry Smoothie ................................ 152
V12 cocktail ................................. 153
Fruity Mint Smoothie ............... 153
Carrot Season ............................. 153
Ringing Red Bell ........................ 154
Carrot & Ginger Cocktail ........ 154
Pineapple Carrot Juice ............ 154
Tomato Fire ................................. 155
Mint, Lime and Cucumber Fresca ................................... 155
Green Tea Smoothie ................ 155
Broccoli, Celery and Kale Juice ............................. 156
Cabbage and Carrot Juice ...... 156
Green Apple Cucumber .......... 156
Berry Green Smoothie ............ 156

Green Life Juice .........................157
Beet It Juice ...............................157
Green Star Smoothie ................157
Broccoli Blast ............................158
Nut Milk 1 ...................................158
Nut Milk 2 ...................................158
Milk of Tahini .............................158
Detox Special ............................159
Green Hemp Milk .....................160
Milk of Tahini .............................160

**Desserts**
French Apple Pie ......................161
Pistachio Halvah.......................161
.Walnut Fudge ...........................162
Pumpkin Pie ..............................162
Coconut-Haystacks .................163
Pecan Pie ...................................163
Strawberry Cream Pie .............164
Almond Smash Macaroons ....165
Cinnamon Ginger Truffles ......165
Persimmon Pie .........................166
Cinnamon Almond Raisin
 Cookies ...................................166
Strawberry Cheesecake ..........167
Orange Sorbet ..........................168
Chocolate Mousse ...................168
Chocolate Avo-Pudding ..........169
Apple Cinnamon Glaze Pie ....170
Cinnamon Glaze ......................170

**Soups**
Herbed Tomato Soup ...............171
Cream of Cucumber Soup .....171
Thai Coconut Soup...................172
Tom kai no-gai ..........................172
Creme of Zucchini....................173
Italian Spinach Soup................173
Cream of Broccoli Soup ..........174
Creamy Avocado Soup ...........175
Cream of Spinach Soup ..........175
Tomato Bisque .........................176

**Breads/Crackers/Crust/Chips**
Pizza Crust ................................177
Onion Bread .............................178
Almond Cinnamon
 Raisin Bread ..........................179
Flax Crackers............................179
Zucchini Bread .........................180
Tortillas......................................180
Veggie Crackers .......................181
Pizza Crackers .........................181
Cheesy Kale Chips ..................182
The Good Cracker ...................183
Kale Chips.................................183
Salt and Vinegar
 Flax Crackers .........................184
Spicy Flax Crackers.................184
Sun-Dried Tomato Crackers ..185
Sun-dried Tomato Olive
 Crackers .................................186
Onion Flax Crackers................186

# Dressings/Sauces/Condiments

### RANCH DRESSING

1 C. pine nuts
¾ C. water
3 Tbs. lemon juice
¼ C. apple cider vinegar
¼ C. extra virgin olive oil
2 cloves garlic
¼ C. chopped onion
1 tsp. dill
⅛ tsp. sea salt
⅛ tsp. ground black pepper

Combine all ingredients and place in blender. Blend and add water slowly until you reach a smooth creamy texture. Store and refrigerate in a glass jar.

### LEMON-BASIL VINAIGRETTE

1 C. extra virgin olive oil
⅓ C. apple cider vinegar
⅛ C. fresh chopped basil
2 cloves garlic
1 Tbs. lemon juice
½ tsp. sea salt

Combine all ingredients and place in a blender and mix. Store and refrigerate in a glass jar.

## CAESAR DRESSING

1 C. pine nuts
½ avocado
¼ C. water
1 Tbs. lemon juice
1 Tbs. Bragg Liquid Aminos
1 clove garlic
¼ tsp. sea salt
⅛ tsp. black pepper

Combine all ingredients in a blender. Blend and add water to reach a creamy texture. Store and refrigerate. Use within 2 days.

## ITALIAN DRESSING

1 C. apple cider vinegar
1 C. extra virgin olive oil
1 Tbs. dried oregano
½ Tbs. garlic powder
½ Tbs. onion powder
½ tsp. dried basil
½ tsp. ground black pepper
¼ tsp. dried thyme
¼ tsp. sea salt

Pour ingredients into a glass jar or bottle with a cover. Cover and shake well. Use or refrigerate.

## MUSTARD

½ C. mustard seeds
1 tsp. turmeric
¾ C. apple cider vinegar
⅓ C. water
½ tsp. lemon juice
¼ tsp. sea salt

Grind mustard seeds. Place all ingredients in a blender. Store and refrigerate in a glass jar.

## GINGER TAHINI MISO DRESSING

⅓ C. Tahini
1 C. water
1 Tbs. white miso
¾ C. Bragg Liquid Aminos
¾ C. scallions
3 Tbs. grated ginger root
3 cloves garlic
½ tsp. ground cumin

Place all ingredients in a blender. Blend and add water to achieve a creamy texture. Store and refrigerate in a glass jar.

## CHIPOTLE SAUCE

2 C. macadamia nuts
1 C. cashews
1 ½ C. water
1 Tbs. lime juice and zest
2 cloves garlic
½ C. lemon juice
1 Tbs. apple cider vinegar
1 chipotle chile
½ tsp. sea salt
½ tsp. stone ground mustard

Combine all ingredients in a blender except water. Blend and add water to reach a creamy texture. Store and refrigerate in a glass jar.

Dressings/Sauces/Condiments

## CHEESE SAUCE

2 C. cashews soaked
1 macadamia nuts soaked
1 C. water
½ C. lemon juice
¼ C. Nama Shoyu or Bragg Liquid Aminos
½ tsp. sea salt

Combine all ingredients in a blender except water. Blend and add water to reach a creamy texture. Store and refrigerate in a glass jar.

## MAYONNAISE

2 C. macadamia nuts
1 ½ C. water
2 cloves garlic
½ C. lemon juice
1 Tbs. apple cider vinegar
½ tsp. sea salt
½ tsp. stone ground mustard

Combine all ingredients in a blender except water. Blend and add water to reach a creamy texture. Store and refrigerate in a glass jar.

## KETCHUP

2 medium tomatoes
1 C. sun dried tomatoes
¼ C. apple cider vinegar
2 Tbs. yacon syrup or ¼ C. soaked dates
1 Tbs. Nama Shoyu or Bragg Liquid Aminos
2 cloves garlic

Place all ingredients in a blender. Blend well. Serve immediately or dehydrate at 115° F for 3 hours. Store in glass jar and refrigerate.

## COCKTAIL SAUCE

6 Tbs. ketchup (see Ketchup Recipe)
¼ C. peeled and cubed horseradish root
¼ C. apple cider vinegar
¼ tsp. sea salt
4 Tbs. lemon juice
⅛ tsp. celery salt

Place horseradish root and apple cider vinegar and salt in a blender. Place blended mixture and all remaining ingredients in a glass jar. Shake well, chill and serve.

## GUACAMOLE

1 avocado
1 small tomato
¼ C. cilantro chopped
¼ C. onion, chopped
2 Tbs. lime juice
1 lemon juice
⅛ tsp. sea salt

Place ingredients in blender and blend.

## SOUR CREAM

1 C. pine nuts
3 Tbs. lemon juice
1 Tbs. Nama Shoyu or Bragg Liquid Aminos
½ C. water

Place ingredients in a blender. Add water and blend until you achieve a creamy texture. Pour into a glass Jar then place a cheese cloth over it and let it sit for 2 hours. Remove cheese cloth and close jar with top and store in the refrigerator.

## SWEET AND SOUR

¼ C. soaked dates
¼ C. apple cider vinegar
¼ C. lemon juice
¼ C. pineapple juice
2 tsp. Nama Shoyu or Bragg Liquid Aminos
¼ C. water

Place ingredients in a blender. Blend until you achieve a smooth texture. Store in a glass jar and refrigerate.

## BBQ SAUCE

2 medium tomatoes
¼ C. chopped onion
½ C. sun dried tomatoes
¼ C. apple cider vinegar
3 Tbs. extra virgin olive oil
2 clove garlic
2 Tbs. yacon syrup or 3 soaked dates
2 tsp. dried oregano
2 tsp. dried thyme
1 Tbs. chili powder

Place all ingredients in a blender. Blend well. Serve immediately or dehydrate at 115° F for 3 hours. Store in glass jar and refrigerate.

## PIZZA SAUCE I

4 medium tomatoes
1 C. extra virgin olive oil
1 red bell pepper
½ medium onion, finely chopped
2 Tbs. parsley, finely chopped
2 Tbs. basil, finely chopped
1 clove garlic
2 Tbs. yacon syrup or 3 soaked dates
1 tsp. sea salt
⅛ tsp. dried red pepper flakes
1 lemon, juiced

Place all ingredients in a blender. Blend well. Serve immediately or dehydrate at 115° F for 4 hours. Store in glass jar and refrigerate.

## PEANUT SAUCE

½ C. coconut milk
½ C. almond butter
3 Tbs. lime juice
1 Tbs. fresh minced ginger
2 Tbs. yacon syrup or 3 soaked dates
¼ C. Nama Shoyu

Place all ingredients except coconut milk in a blender. Blend ingredients and slowly add coconut milk until you achieve a creamy texture. Store and refrigerate in a glass jar.

# CHEDDAR CHEESE SAUCE

1 C. soaked cashews
3 Tbs. lemon juice
1 small red bell pepper
1 C. water
2 Tbs. extra virgin olive oil
3 tsp. Nama Shoyu or Bragg Liquid Aminos
1 tsp. sea salt
1 tsp. habanero chili, chopped

Place ingredients in a blender. Add water and blend until you achieve a creamy texture. Pour into a glass jar then place a cheese cloth over it and let it sit for 2 hours. Remove cheese cloth and close jar with top and store in the refrigerator.

# SOUR CREAM AND ONION DIP

1 C. sour cream (see Sour Cream recipe)
½ C. minced onion
1 Tbs. brown miso
¼ tsp. celery seed

In a bowl add minced onion, brown miso, and celery seed to sour cream recipe and mix thoroughly.

# PAD THAI SAUCE

½ C. warm water
¼ C. dates
½ C. of prunes or apricots
2 Tbs. lime
1 tsp. dried crushed chili or cayenne pepper

Place all ingredients in blender and blend.

## SALSA

2 tomatoes
¼ red onion
¼ C. scallions
½ yellow bell pepper
¼ C. cilantro
3 Tbs. lime juice
1 Tbs. lemon juice
⅛ tsp. sea salt

## VINAIGRETTE

1 C. extra virgin olive oil
½ C. apple cider vinegar
1 bunch shallot, minced
1 tsp. chopped fresh thyme
1 Tbs. mustard (see Mustard recipe)
⅛ tsp. sea salt

Place ingredients in a blender and blend.

## PESTO

2 C. fresh basil leaves, packed
½ C. cheese sauce
½ C. extra virgin olive oil
⅓ C. pine nuts or walnuts
3 garlic cloves, minced
⅛ tsp. sea salt
⅛ tsp. ground black pepper

Place ingredients in a food processor and pulse until you see it is well blended.

## LEMON VINAIGRETTE DRESSING

½ C. extra virgin olive oil
1 tsp. finely shredded lemon peel
⅓ C. lemon juice
3 cloves garlic, minced
⅛ tsp. sea salt
⅛ tsp. ground black pepper

Pour ingredients into a glass jar or bottle with a cover. Cover and shake well. Use or refrigerate.

## CAESAR DRESSING IHI

2 avocados
⅓ C. lemon juice
1 Tbs. black pepper
½ Tbs. salt
1 tsp. cayenne
3 Tbs. extra virgin olive oil
¼ C. water

Place all ingredients in a blender. Add water until you reach a creamy texture. Serve immediately.

## RICOTTA CHEESE

2 C. cashews soaked
2 C. macadamia nuts soaked
1 C. water
½ C. lemon juice
½ C. Nama Shoyu or Bragg Liquid Aminos
½ tsp. sea salt

Combine all ingredients in a blender or food processor. Mix and add water slowly to reach a fluffy texture. Store in a glass jar or container.

## CHOW MEIN SAUCE

1 Tbs. almond butter
2 Tbs. Nama Shoyu
¾ tsp. onion powder
½ tsp. powdered ginger
2 cloves garlic minced
⅛ tsp. sea salt
⅛ tsp. ground black pepper

Combine all ingredients in a blender and blend. Store in a glass jar.

## MUSHROOM GRAVY

1 C. portobello mushrooms sliced
2 Tbs. dark miso
2 C. warm to hot water

Place miso in a bowl, add water and mix well. Decrease or add water to make gravy thick or thin. Add in sliced mushrooms. Serve warm.

# Salads

## KALE SALAD WITH PINE NUTS, APRICOTS, AND CHEESE SAUCE

¼ C. apricots chopped
2 bunches of kale
1 Tbs. extra virgin olive oil
2 Tbs. pine nuts
½ tsp. sea salt
2 Tbs. cheese sauce

Remove leaves from stem and center ribs. Cut leaves into thin strips. Place all ingredients into a bowl and toss thoroughly. Serve and enjoy!

## THAI TOMATO SALAD

1 container of cherry or grape tomatoes
1 cucumber
1 red bell pepper
½ red onion

Chop all ingredients and place in a salad bowl. Top with Ginger Tahini Miso Dressing.

## GREEN HOUSE SALAD

1 head of green leaf lettuce
1 cucumber
1 red bell pepper
½ red onion
1 container of cherry or grape tomatoes
1 stalk of celery

Chop all ingredients except tomatoes and place in a salad bowl. Top with Italian Dressing.

## TACO SALAD

3 leaves of green leaf lettuce
2 Tbs. taco meat (see Taco Meat recipe)
3 Tbs. guacamole
2 Tbs. salsa
2 Tbs. sour cream

Chop lettuce and top it with taco meat, guacamole, salsa, and sour cream.

## CAESAR SALAD

1 head romaine lettuce chopped
1 large carrot shredded
5 cherry tomatoes diced
½ C. dried coconut grated

Combine ingredients in a bowl and add Caesar Dressing. Toss well and serve.

## SPINACH SALAD WITH RED ONION AND HAZELNUTS

8 C. baby spinach leaves
1 C. thinly sliced red onion
⅔ C. hazelnuts, chopped

Place hazelnuts in a food processor or blender and process until they are chopped. Place all ingredients in a bowl. Pair with Lemon Basil Vinaigrette Dressing.

## FARMER'S SALAD

½ pound squash halved
½ pound green beans trimmed
8 C. mixed salad greens
⅓ C. fresh basil leaves
1 container grape or cherry tomatoes
½ C. black olives

Chop ingredients and combine in a bowl. Pair with Vinaigrette Dressing.

## TOMATO-RADICCHIO WITH BASIL VINAIGRETTE

⅓ C. chopped fresh basil
8 whole large basil leaves
3 Tbs. extra-virgin olive oil
2 Tbs. apple cider vinegar
8 radicchio leaves, thick ends trimmed
2 large tomatoes, peeled, halved, thinly sliced

Place ingredients in a bowl. Serve with Lemon Basil Vinaigrette.

## CANDIED WALNUT SALAD

12 oz. walnut halves
1 C. extra virgin olive oil
½ C. apple cider vinegar
2 Tbs. chopped fresh chives
2 Tbs. chopped fresh parsley or chervil
2 Tbs. yacon syrup
1 tsp. cinnamon
1 ¼ tsp. chopped fresh dill
10 oz. arugula leaves or spring mix
sea salt to taste

Place walnuts, yacon syrup, and cinnamon in a bowl and mix. Place mixture on dehydrator tray and dehydrate at 115° F for 3 hours. Combine olive oil, vinegar, chives, parsley or chervil, dill, and salt in a glass jar. Mix well. Place arugula leaves or spring mix, candied walnuts, and dressing in a bowl. Toss and enjoy!

## CURRY CABBAGE SALAD

1 head green cabbage, chopped
⅓ C. shredded carrot
2 Tbs. lemon juice
¼ C. extra virgin olive oil
¼ C. Nama Shoyu or Bragg Liquid Aminos
3 Tbs. sesame seeds
⅓ tsp. turmeric
½ tsp. curry
½ tsp. cumin

Place all ingredients in a bowl. Mix well and serve.

## PAD THAI SALAD

2 zucchinis, sliced thin
2 C. mung bean sprouts
¾ C. almonds or cashews
1 red bell pepper, sliced into strips
2 green onions, diced
1 Tbs. lime juice
1 Tbs. extra virgin olive oil
⅛ tsp. sea salt

## COLE SLAW

2 C. cabbage shredded
¼ C. onion shredded
1 C. carrot shredded
¼ C. green onion thinly sliced
¼ C. mayonnaise

Place all ingredients in a bowl. Mix well and serve.

## ITALIAN PESTO SALAD

2 C. romaine lettuce - torn, washed and dried
1 C. torn escarole
1 C. torn radicchio
1 C. torn red leaf lettuce
¼ C. chopped green onions
½ red bell pepper, sliced into rings
½ yellow bell pepper, sliced in rings
1 container cherry or grape tomatoes
¼ C. pesto
¼ C. extra virgin olive oil
2 Tbs. lemon juice
⅛ tsp. sea salt
⅛ tsp. pepper

Place all ingredients in a bowl. Mix well and serve.

## TOMATO BASIL SALAD

1 head of green leaf lettuce, torn
2 Tbs. extra virgin olive oil
2 cloves garlic, minced
3 C. fresh basil, torn
1 container grape or cherry tomatoes, halved
½ C. pine nuts
3 Tbs. cheese sauce

Place all ingredients in a bowl and mix well. Pair with Lemon Vinaigrette Dressing.

## BROCCOLI SALAD

6 C. broccoli florets
½ C. slivered almonds
½ C. eggplant bacon
¼ red onion, chopped
1 C. peas
½ C. mayonnaise
2 Tbs. apple cider vinegar
½ tsp. sea salt

Place all ingredients in a bowl. Mix well. Refrigerate or serve immediately.

## CHERRY TOMATO CUCUMBER SALAD

- 3 C. of cherry, grape, or pear tomatoes, sliced in half
- 1 C. of chopped cucumber, peeled
- ¼ C. cheese sauce
- 1 Tbsp mint leaves cut into thin strips
- 1 tsp. oregano
- 1 Tbs. lemon juice
- 2 Tbs. of finely chopped green onions
- 2 tsp. extra virgin olive oil
- ⅛ tsp. sea salt
- ⅛ tsp. ground black pepper

Place all ingredients in a bowl. Mix well and serve.

## CARROT SALAD

- 4 C. grated carrots
- 1 C. raisins
- 1 large apple, cored and chopped
- ⅓ C. mayonnaise

Place all ingredients in a bowl. Mix well and serve.

## CUCUMBER SALAD

- 2 large cucumbers peeled, quartered lengthwise, then sliced crosswise
- 2 Tbs. chopped fresh dill or basil
- 3 Tbs. apple cider vinegar
- ⅛ tsp. sea salt
- ⅛ tsp. ground black pepper

Place all ingredients in a bowl. Mix well and serve.

## JICAMA SALAD

- 1 large jicama peeled, then cubed
- ½ red bell pepper, finely diced
- ½ yellow bell pepper, finely diced
- ½ green bell pepper, finely diced
- ½ C. chopped red onion
- ½ large cucumber, seeded, chopped
- ½ C. chopped fresh cilantro
- ⅓ C. lime juice
- ⅛ tsp. sea salt
- ⅛ tsp. paprika
- Pinch of cayenne

Place all ingredients in a bowl. Mix well, let chill for 30 minutes, then serve.

## SEAWEED AND KALE SALAD

½ C. dried wakame seaweed
1 Tbs. Tahini
1 Tbs. peeled and minced ginger
1 bunch kale
2 clove garlic, minced
2 Tbs. Bragg Liquid Aminos
1 Tbs. sesame seeds

Rinse and soak kale and seaweed in warm water for 5 minutes. Drain seaweed and place in a bowl. Drain kale and chop into thin slices. Place all ingredients in a bowl and mix well. Toss and serve.

## MAKE IT WORK SALAD

Use your favorite veggies, pates, nuts and seeds.

Chop, shred, grind, and combine all in a bowl. Mix well and serve with your favorite dressing. Enjoy!

# Breakfast

## PECAN PORRIDGE

1 C. pecans
2 Tbs. yacon syrup
1 Tbs. extra virgin olive oil
1 tsp. cinnamon
⅛ tsp. sea salt
8 oz. warm to hot water

Place all ingredients in a blender. Add water until you reach the desired consistency.

## PECAN AND BLUEBERRY PORRIDGE

1 C. pecans
½ C. blueberries
2 Tbs. yacon syrup
1 Tbs. extra virgin olive oil
1 tsp. cinnamon
⅛ tsp. sea salt
8 oz. warm to hot water

Place all ingredients in a blender. Add water until you reach the desired consistency.

## MACADAMIA NUT PORRIDGE

Pulp of 4 young coconuts
½ C. macadamia nuts, unsoaked
½ vanillla bean
Pinch of Celtic salt

Blend and serve.

## GRANOLA

1 C. almonds, soaked
1 C. sunflower seeds, soaked
½ C. walnuts, soaked
½ C. pecans, soaked
½ C. pumpkin seeds, soaked
4 Tbs. yacon syrup
1 Tbs. coconut cream
1 tsp. cinnamon
1 tsp. vanilla
1 tsp. nutmeg
½ tsp. salt

Place all ingredients in a food processor and pulse to achieve a chopped texture. Spoon out mixture onto a mesh dehydrator sheet. Spread out mixture to ¼ inch thickness and dehydrate at 115° F for 12 hours. Serve with nut milk and eat as a cereal or break off and eat as a snack.

## BUCKWHEAT GRANOLA

3 C. buckwheat, soaked
1 C. almonds, soaked
1 apple, cored and chopped
1 tsp. ginger powder
½ C. pumpkin seed, soaked
2 tsp. vanilla extract
2 tsp. pumpkin pie spice
4 Tbs. yacon syrup
¼ C. raisins

Place all ingredients in a food processor and pulse to achieve a chopped texture. Spoon out mixture onto a mesh dehydrator sheet. Spread out mixture to ¼ inch thickness and dehydrate at 115° F for 12 hours. Serve with nut milk and eat as a cereal or break off and eat as a snack.

# LIVING BAGEL

1 C. almonds, ground or almond pulp
½ C. sunflower seeds
1 cup carrot pulp
⅛ tsp. sea salt
2 Tbs. olive oil
1 cup flax, ground
1 zucchini, shredded

Grind sunflower seeds and flax seeds into flour with a coffee grinder or food processor. Put flax and sunflower flour and remaining ingredients in a food processor and mix thoroughly. Take 2 tablespoons of mixture and shape into a round ball and flatten it onto Teflex sheet and spread it out to have a ½ inch thickness. Dehydrate at 115° F for 6 hours and then flip bagels onto a mesh dehydrator tray and dehydrate at 115° F for an additional 6 hours.

# Entrees

## PIZZA (MAKES 1 PIZZA CRUST)

2 C. ground sunflower seeds
2 C. ground flax seed
1 small tomato
¼ red onion
¼ C. extra virgin olive oil
½ C. water
½ tsp. salt
½ tsp. thyme

Put all ingredients in a food processor to mix thoroughly to form a dough. You can add more water for doughy consistency. Form into the shape of a pizza by molding with your hands. Dehydrate at 100° for 12 hours.

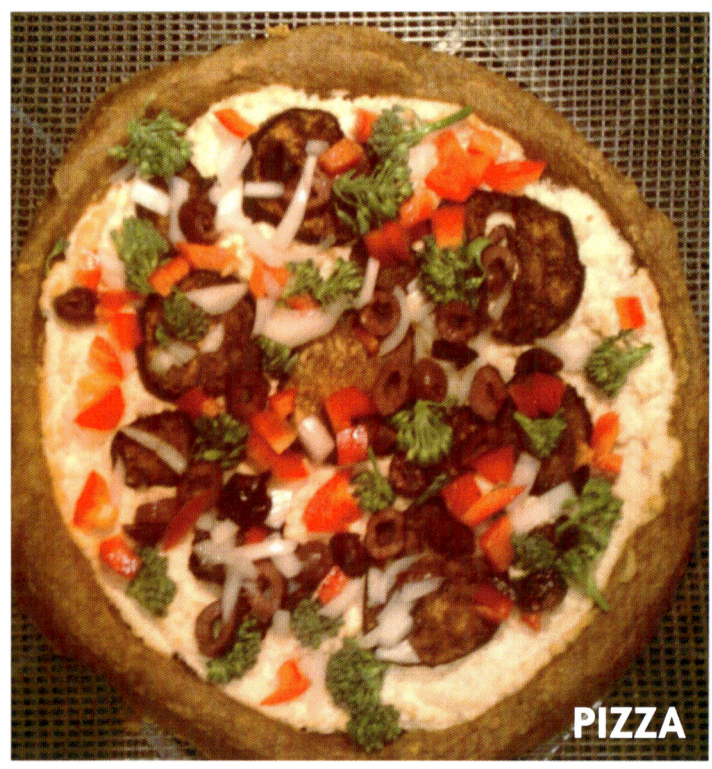

## CHEEZE

2 C. cashews, soaked bunch cilantro
1 C. macadamia nuts, soaked
2 Tbs. lemon juice
¼ C. Nama Shoyu
¼ C. water

Put all ingredients in a food processor to mix thoroughly until it becomes creamy.

## PIZZA SAUCE II

3 medium tomatoes
¼ bunch basil
2 C. sun dried tomatoes
¼ C. water
¼ C. olive oil
2 clove garlic
2 Tbs. oregano
2 Tbs. thyme
½ tsp. salt
1 lemon, juiced
1 date

Toppings:
¼ C. broccoli florets
¼ C. Kalamata olives
½ onion, sliced thin
1 medium tomato, sliced
½ C. pineapple chunks
½ tsp. salt

Spread pizza sauce around the inner crust. Then spread cheeze over pizza sauce. Then add toppings. Dehydrate for 4 hours at 115° F. Serve and enjoy!

## TACO

8 Leaves of Romaine lettuce

Taco Meat:
1 C. almonds
1 C. walnuts
1 clove garlic
1 Tbs. season all
2 Tbs. taco seasoning
2 Tbs. Bragg Liquid Aminos
¼ C. extra virgin olive oil

Place all ingredients in a food processor. Process until well mixed and nuts become a consistency of pate. You can dehydrate at 115° F for 4 hours or serve as is.

Put taco meat inside of lettuce and top with salsa, guacamole, nacho cheese and sour cream.

## SPRING ROLLS

2 heads of white cabbage
1 C. walnuts, soaked
1 C. almonds, soaked
½ C. pine nuts, unsoaked
1 large carrot, finely chopped
1 bell pepper, finely chopped
½ C. olive oil
½ C. water
1 tsp. cayenne
1 Tbs. marjoram
1 Tbs. sage
1 Tbs. thyme
1 tsp. fresh ginger, finely chopped
1 ½ Tbs. Celtic salt

Soak cabbage head in warm water for 20 minutes. Place all ingredients except cabbage head in a food processor and mix until smooth. Mix remaining ingredients together and knead into the nut mixture. Spoon the nut mixture into the cabbage leaves. Carefully tuck the ends and roll it into a spring roll.

# MASSAMAN

- 1 C. yellow squash, cut into chunks
- 14 oz. coconut milk
- ½ C. warm water
- 1 small red pepper, thinly sliced
- 1 medium tomato, sliced
- 2 Tbs. extra virgin olive oil
- ⅓ C. onion, sliced
- 1 thumb-piece ginger, grated
- 4 cloves garlic
- ¾ tsp. chili powder/cayenne pepper
- 1 Tbs. brown miso
- 1 stalk lemongrass, minced
- 1 tsp. turmeric
- ¼ C. chopped raw cashews
- ¼ C. cilantro
- 1 tsp. cumin
- ½ tsp. pepper
- ⅛ tsp. ginger
- 4 dates
- 1 Tbs. lime juice
- 1 head of broccoli
- 1 carrot sliced thin

Place dates, brown miso, lime juice and ½ cup of warm water in a blender and mix well, then join all ingredients together in a bowl and mix well. Serve warm.

## TEMPURA VEGETABLES

4 C. broccoli tops
1 C. cauliflower
½ C. pistachios, unsoaked
1 C. pine nuts, unsoaked
½ C. lemon juice
3 tsp. Celtic salt
½ C. olive oil
1 C. water

Place pistachios, pine nuts, salt, lemon, and olive oil in a blender. Slowly add water until you achieve a smooth consistency. Place vegetables in bowl, add sauce, and mix thoroughly. Spoon vegetables onto Teflex sheets on dehydrator trays and dehydrate for 3 hours at 115° degrees. Serve warm.

## LIFE BURGERS

1 C. almonds
1 C. walnuts
½ medium tomato
2 Tbs. dark miso
½ C. oregano chopped
½ yellow onion
2 cloves garlic, minced
½ C. olive oil
2 tsp. paprika
1 tsp. thyme
1 tsp. sea salt

Place all ingredients in a food processor. Process until well mixed and nuts become a consistency of pate. Dehydrate at 115° F for 4 hours or serve as is.

# LIVING LIFE EGGPLANT "BACON" BURGERS

1 C. almonds
1 C. walnuts
½ C. sunflower seeds
8 strips "eggplant bacon"
2 C. portobello mushrooms, chopped
½ yellow onion
2 C. chopped celery,
6 C. garlic
¼ C. extra virgin olive oil
¼ C. Nama Shoyu or Bragg Liquid Aminos
Several slices of onion bread

Place all ingredients except onion bread and eggplant bacon in a food processor. Process until nuts become a consistency of pate. Dehydrate at 115° F for 4 hours or serve as is. Place burgers on onion bread and top with lettuce, tomato, onion, ketchup, eggplant bacon, and mustard.

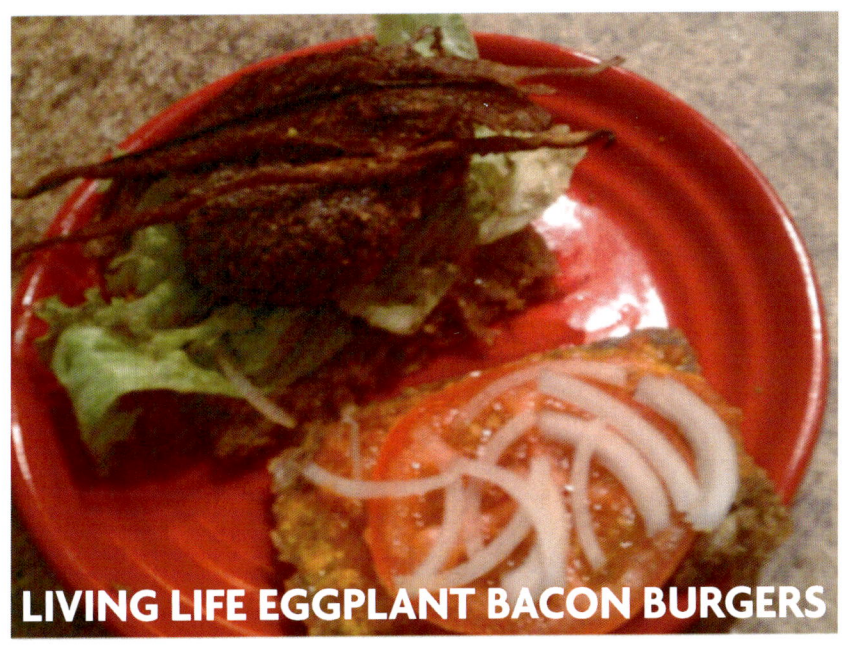

LIVING LIFE EGGPLANT BACON BURGERS

# CHESAPEAKE BAY NORI ROLLS

1 crab cake recipe (see page
½ cucumber, sliced thin like sticks
2 carrots, shredded
1 ricotta cheese recipe (see page
1 pack of enoki mushrooms
1 avocado, sliced into chunks
1 red bell pepper, sliced into strips

On a sheet of nori spread out the crab cake mixture over ⅓ of the sheet. Layer it with avocado, several enoki mushrooms, shredded carrots, and red bell pepper. Roll up the nori roll and slice into 4 to 6 pieces with a slightly wet knife. Serve with Nama Shoyu or Bragg Liquid Aminos.

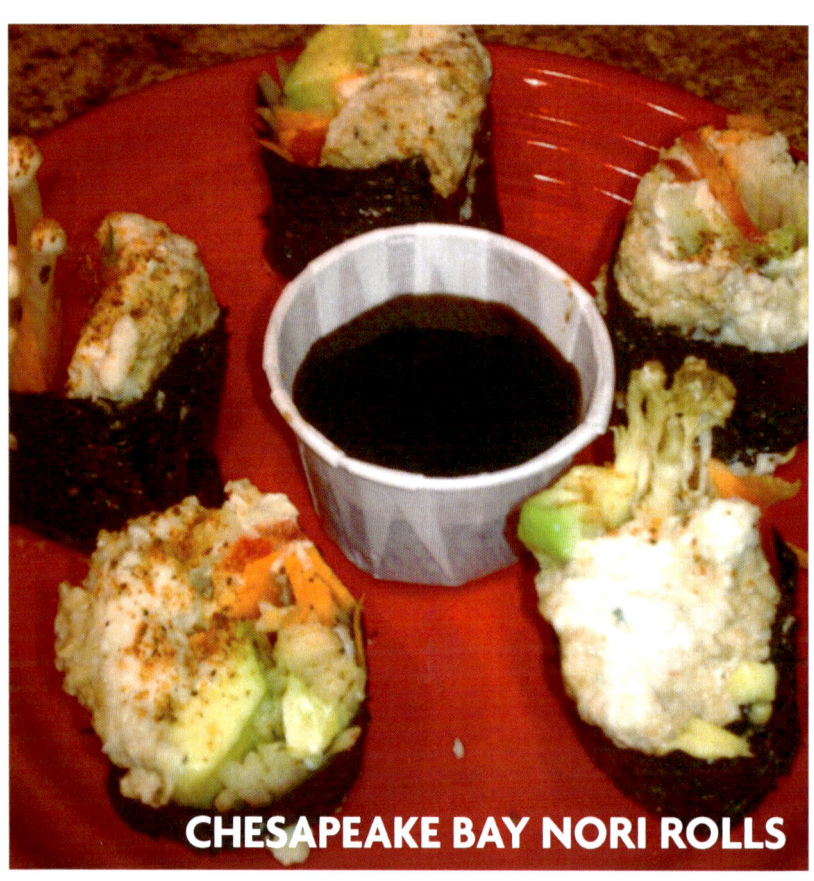

# CREATING CHEESAPEAKE BAY NORI ROLLS

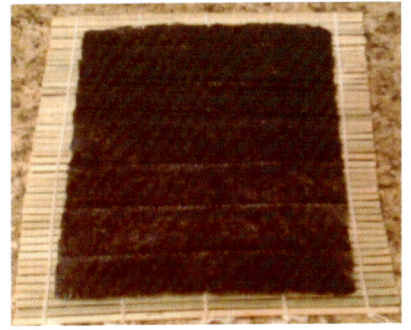
Step 1

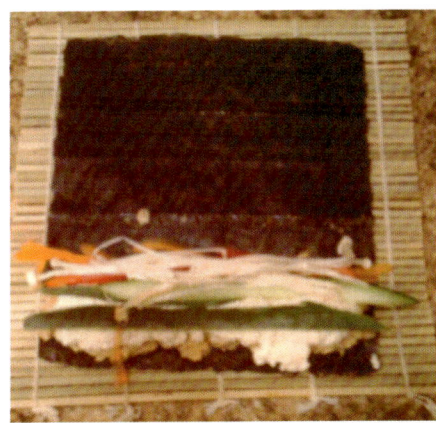
Step 2

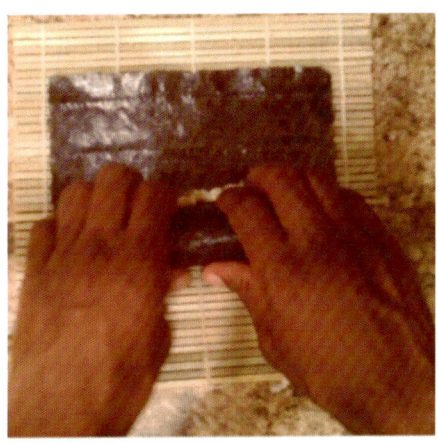
Step 3

Step 4

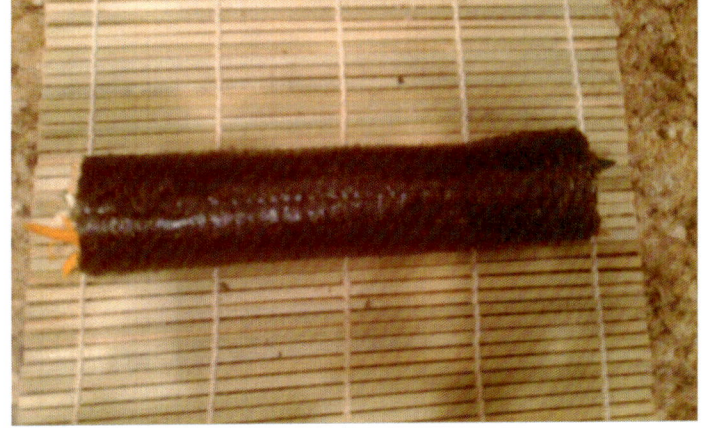

## LASAGNA

4 zucchini, sliced long, flat, and ¼ inch thick
1 recipe life burger
1 recipe ricotta
1 recipe pizza sauce
2 medium tomatoes, sliced ⅛ inch thick

Lay 4 slices of zucchini side by side in a glass baking dish. Cover evenly with life burger, followed by ricotta, then pizza sauce. Place another layer of zucchini on top. Cover evenly with ricotta, sliced tomatoes, and another layer of pizza sauce. Dehydrate at 145° F for 3 hours. Reduce to 115° F for 6 to 8 hours or serve immediately.

## PASTA MARINARA OR PESTO

6 zucchini, peeled and cut like spaghetti with a spiral slicer. Or use 2 packs of kelp noodles, soaked
1 recipe of pizza sauce or pesto sauce

Place zucchini or kelp noodles in a bowl and pour sauce over the noodles and mix well. Dehydrate at 115° F for 5 hours or serve immediately.

## CHOW MEIN

1 recipe chow mein sauce
3 C. mung bean sprouts
1 recipe cole slaw
10 snow peas
1 red bell pepper, cut in thin strips
3 scallions or chives, cut into long pieces

Place veggies in a bowl and mix well with chow mein sauce.

## CHIPOTLE LIME TACOS

8 pieces of Romaine lettuce
1 C. cherry tomatoes, sliced in halves
½ C. sprouts (broccoli, alfalfa, etc.)
1 avocado, sliced thin
2 Tbs. chipotle sauce (see Chipotle recipe)
1 Tbs. lime juice

Place sprouts, tomatoes, and avocado inside of Romaine lettuce. Top with chipotle sauce and sprinkle tacos with lime juice.

## TUNA SALAD

2 C. sunflower seeds
3 stalks celery, diced
¼ yellow onion
½ bunch scallions, chopped
2 Tbs. dulse flakes
½ C. dried dill
1 tsp. sea salt
⅛ tsp. black pepper
½ C. mayonnaise (see Mayonnaise recipe)

Place all ingredients in a food processor and mix thoroughly.

## SLOPPY JOE

2 crumbled burgers (see Burger recipes)
1 C. pizza sauce
1 Tbs. chili powder
2 tsp. apple cider vinegar
Several slices of onion bread (see Onion Bread recipe)
2 C. lettuce, shredded

Place all ingredients except lettuce and onion bread in a bowl and mix thoroughly. Place sloppy joe mixture on a slice of onion bread and top with lettuce and the other piece of onion bread. Enjoy!

## CHICKEN SALAD

2 C. sunflower seeds
1 stalk celery, diced
¼ medium yellow onion
½ bunch scallions, chopped
2 Tbs. parsley, chopped
¼ C. dried dill
1 tsp. sea salt
⅛ tsp. black pepper
½ C. mayonnaise (see Mayonnaise recipe)

Place all ingredients in a food processor and mix thoroughly.

## CRAB CAKES

C. sunflower seeds
⅓ C. ground almonds unsoaked
3 green onions (green and white parts), finely chopped
½ C. finely chopped red bell pepper
½ C. mayonnaise recipe
1 tsp. ground mustard seed
1 Tbs. lemon juice
2 cloves garlic, minced
1 tsp. sea salt
2 Tbs. Old Bay seasoning

Place all ingredients in a food processor and mix thoroughly. Form into patties and dehydrate at 115° F for 4 hours or serve immediately. Serve with cocktail sauce.

# EGGPLANT BACON

1 eggplant, sliced long ⅛ inch thick
¼ C. extra virgin olive oil
1 Tbs. ground fennel

Marinate eggplant in olive oil and fennel for 4 hours. Place on mesh dehydrator sheets at 115° F for 12 hours.

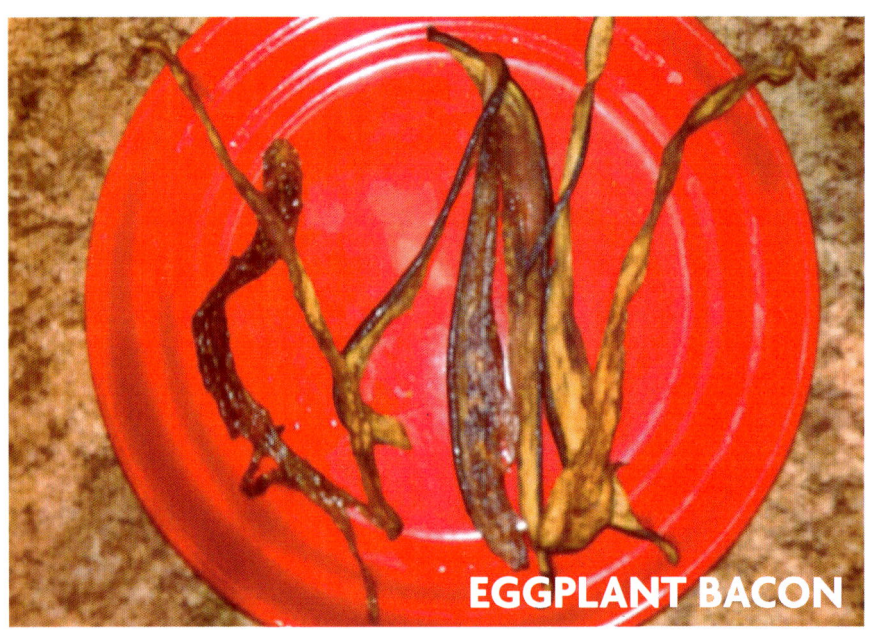

# VEGGIE FAJITAS

2 portobello mushrooms, sliced
3 red and or yellow bell peppers, sliced into strips
1 zucchini, sliced into strips
1 red onion, thinly sliced
2 cloves garlic, minced
¼ C. Nama Shoyu or Bragg Liquid Aminos
¼ C. extra virgin olive oil
1 ½ Tbs. chili powder
1 tsp. cumin
¼ tsp. cayenne
1 Tbs. apple cider vinegar

Place all ingredients in a bowl and mix together thoroughly. Let marinate for 2-6 hours. Dehydrate for 4 hours or use immediately. Place marinated veggies in lettuce and top with sour cream, salsa, guacamole, and cheese sauce. Enjoy!

# SPINACH LASAGNA

4 zucchini, sliced long, flat, and ¼ inch thick
2 medium tomatoes, sliced ⅛ inch thick
handful of spinach, chopped

Lay 4 slices of zucchini side by side in a glass baking dish. Cover evenly ricotta, spinach, then pizza sauce. Place another layer of zucchini on top. Cover evenly with ricotta, sliced tomatoes, and another layer of pizza sauce. Dehydrate at 145° F for 3 hours Reduce to 115° F for 6 to 8 hours or serve immediately.

Pizza Sauce #3
4 medium tomatoes
½ C. extra virgin olive oil
½ medium onion, finely chopped
2 Tbs. basil, finely chopped
1 clove garlic
1 tsp. sea salt
1 Tbs. dried red pepper flakes
1 lemon, juiced

Place all ingredients in a blender. Blend well. Serve immediately or dehydrate at 115° F for 4 hours.

Ricotta Cheese #2
1 C. cashews soaked
1 C. water
½ C. lemon juice
½ C. Nama Shoyu or Bragg Liquid Aminos
½ tsp. sea salt

Combine all ingredients in a blender or food processor. Mix and add water slowly to reach a fluffy texture.

# Entrees

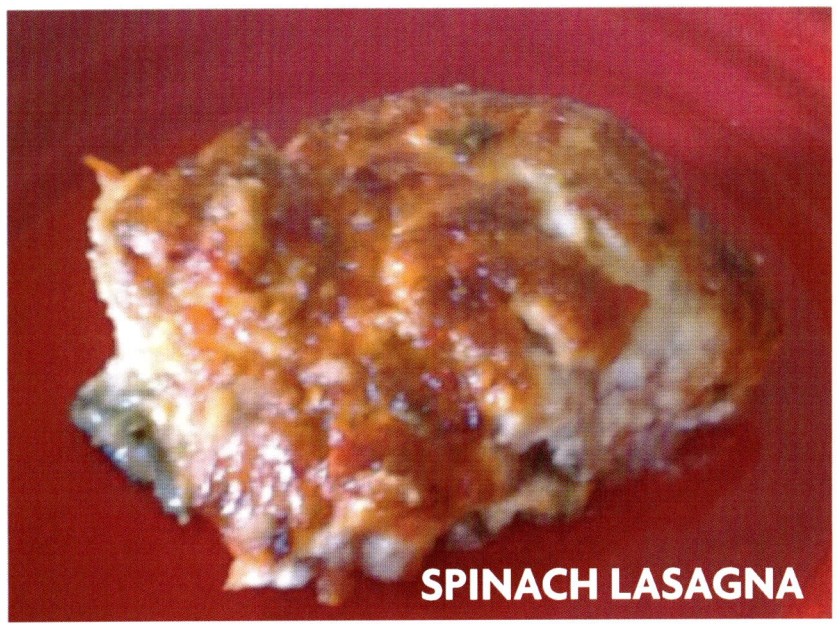

SPINACH LASAGNA

## STUFFED BELL PEPPERS

4 bell peppers, red, yellow, or orange
1 tsp. sea salt
5 Tbs. extra-virgin olive oil
1 medium yellow onion, chopped
1 taco meat recipe
1 ½ C "rice" recipe
1 C. tomatoes chopped
1 Tbs. oregano, chopped
Fresh ground pepper
½ C. Ketchup recipe
½ tsp. Nama Shoyu
⅛ tsp. Tabasco sauce

Place all ingredients except bell peppers in a bowl and mix together. Prepare bell peppers by cutting off the tops and removing the inner core and pith. Stuff the bell peppers with the filling. Dehydrate at 145° F for 2 hours.

# Snacks/Appetizers

## RED BELL PEPPER HUMMUS

4 zucchini
½ C. tahini
1 clove garlic, minced
1 tsp. ground cumin
½ tsp. ground coriander
½ red bell pepper
1 Tbs. white miso
2 tsp. apple cider vinegar
1 Tbs. olive oil
¼ tsp. sea salt
⅛ tsp. ground pepper

Place all ingredients in a food processor and mix until you achieve a smooth creamy consistency. Serve and enjoy.

## HUMMUS

4 zucchini
¾ C. tahini
½ C. lemon juice
¼ C. extra virgin olive oil
2 cloves garlic
1 tsp. sea salt
¾ Tbs. ground cumin

Place all ingredients in a blender and blend until you reach a thick and creamy texture.

## EGG-LESS SALAD

1 C. macadamia nuts
½ C. water
½ C. lemon juice
2 cloves garlic
¼ C. scallions, chopped
¼ C. celery, chopped
½ red bell pepper
2 tsp. turmeric
1 tsp. sea salt

Place macadamia nuts, lemon juice, water, red bell pepper, turmeric, and sea salt in a blender and blend until smooth and creamy. Place mixture in a bowl and add in scallions and celery. Mix well and serve.

## MASHED POTATOES

2 C. cauliflower
¼ C. macadamia nuts
¼ C. pine nuts
¼ C. extra virgin olive oil
2 cloves garlic
1 tsp. sea salt
⅛ tsp. ground black pepper
¼ C. chives

Place all ingredients except pepper and chives in a food processor and mix until it becomes smooth and fluffy. Top with pepper and chives. Serve with mushroom gravy.

## "RICE"

- 4 parsnips, peeled and roughly chopped
- 2 ½ Tbs. tahini
- 2 Tbs. Nama Shoyu or Bragg Liquid Aminos
- 1 tsp. extra virgin olive oil
- 2 tsp. apple cider vinegar
- ⅛ tsp. sea salt
- ⅛ tsp. pepper

Place ingredients in a food processor and pulse until it reaches the consistency of rice. Use in other dishes such as nori rolls or as a dish with mushroom gravy. Enjoy!

## ZUCCHINI FRIES

- 2 zucchini, sliced in the shape of fries
- ¼ tsp. garlic powder
- ¼ tsp. dried basil
- 2 Tbs. extra virgin olive oil
- ⅛ tsp. sea salt

Place all ingredients in a bowl. Toss and mix thoroughly. Place zucchini fries on a mesh dehydrator tray and dehydrate at 115° F for 10 hours or until crispy. Serve with ketchup and mustard.

# TOMATO CHIPS

2 tomatos, sliced
1/8 tsp. sea salt
1 Tbs. extra virgin olive oil

Take tomatoes and slice ¼ inch thick and place in a bowl with remaining ingredients. Toss and mix thoroughly. Place tomatoes on a mesh dehydrator tray and dehydrate at 115° F for 10 hours until crispy.

# Juices/Smoothies/Milks

## BLOOD ORANGE CHRISTIAN

1 blood orange
1 cucumber, peeled
1 C. tomato juice, chilled
¼ C. lemon juice
1 Tbs. hot sauce

Place all ingredients in a blender and blend well. Strain juice into a glass, add celery stalk and serve immediately.

## BANANA BREAKFAST SHAKE

2 ripe bananas
¼ C. cashew
½ C. nut milk (almond, brazil, etc)
½ tsp. vanilla extract

Place all ingredients in a blender and blend until smooth. Serve immediately.

## ALMOND & BANANA SMOOTHIE

½ C. almonds
2 C. nut milk (almond, brazil, etc)
2 ripe bananas, halved
1 tsp. vanilla extract
⅛ tsp. ground cinnamon

Place almonds in a blender and blend until finely chopped. Add milk, bananas, and vanilla and blend until creamy and smooth. Pour into a glass and sprinkle with cinnamon.

## PINEAPPLE MELON SMOOTHIE

½ C. pineapple juice
¼ C. orange juice
4 C. honey dew melon, cut into chunks
1 C. frozen pineapple chunks
4 ice cubes, crushed

Place all ingredients in a blender and blend until you reach a slushy consistency. Pour mix into a glass and serve.

## ORANGE AND RED KICKER

1 C. carrot juice
1 C. tomato juice
2 large red, yellow, or orange bell pepper, deseeded and coarsely chopped.
1 tsp. lemon juice
1 tsp. ground black pepper

Place all ingredients in a blender and blend well. Pour into a glass and serve.

## BITTER SWEET BEET SMOOTHIE

1 C. freshly squeezed orange juice
¼ C. beet juice
¼ C. cashew
⅔ C. water
1 C. ice

Place all ingredients in a blender and blend well. Pour into a glass and serve.

# TROPICAL STRAWBERRY SMOOTHIE

1 ½ C. strawberry, stemmed
½ C. pineapple chunks
½ C. orange juice
1 ½ C. ice

Place all ingredients in a blender and blend well. Pour into a glass and serve.

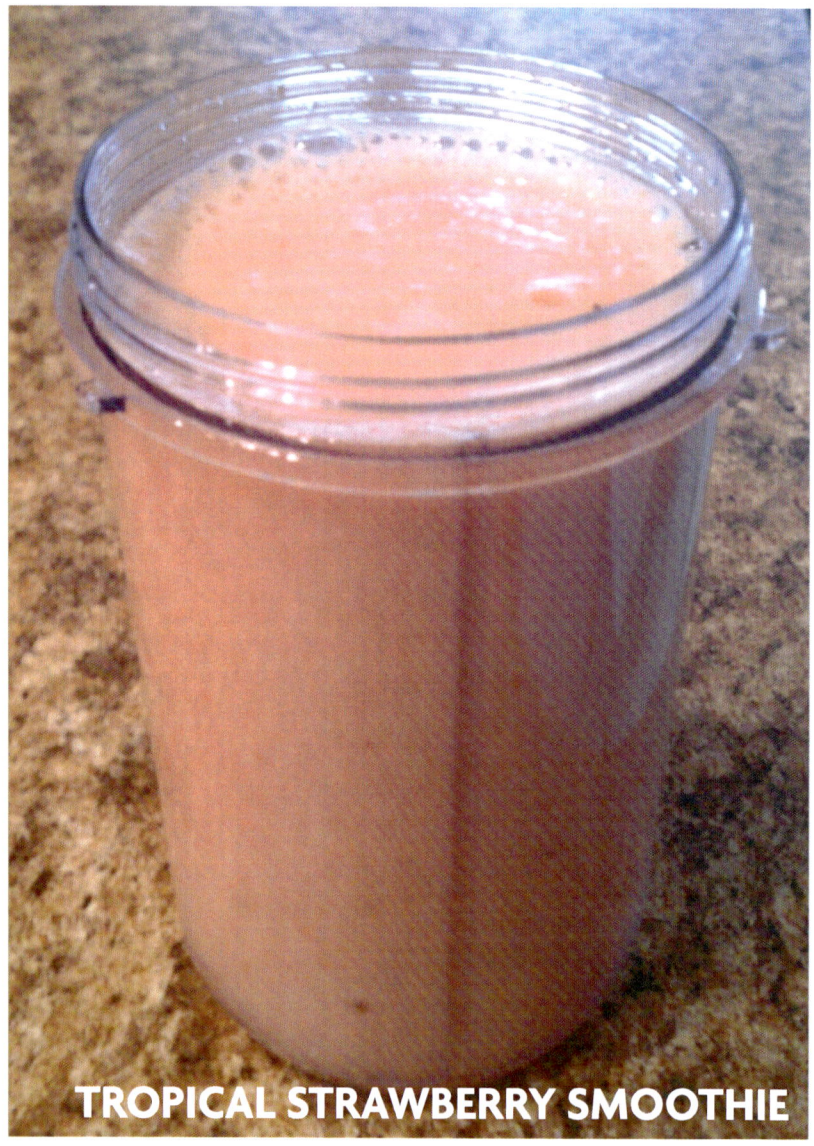

# V12 COCKTAIL

½ C. carrot juice
2 tomatoes, skinned, deseeded, and coarsely chopped
1 Tbs. lemon juice
4 celery stalks, trimmed and sliced
4 scallions, trimmed and coarsely chopped
⅓ C. parsley
⅓ C. mint

Place all ingredients in a blender and blend until smooth. Pour into a glass and serve.

# FRUITY MINT SMOOTHIE

2 C. mango flesh
4 C. kiwi flesh
1 C. pineapple, sliced
4 fresh mint leaves

Place all ingredients in a blender and blend well. Serve over ice and enjoy!

# CARROT SEASON

½ C. carrot
1 C. pineapple, sliced
1 Tbs. lemon juice

Place all ingredients in a blender and blend. Serve over ice and enjoy.

## RINGING RED BELL

1 C. carrot juice
1 C. tomato juice
2 large red bell peppers, seeded and coarsely chopped
1 Tbs. lemon juice
⅛ tsp. ground black pepper

Place all ingredients in a blender and blend well. Serve over ice and enjoy.

## CARROT & GINGER COCKTAIL

1 C. carrot juice
4 tomatoes, skinned, deseeded, and coarsely chopped
1 ripe banana
1 Tbs. lemon juice
⅓ C. parsley
¼ ginger
2 ice cubes, crushed
½ cup water

Place all ingredients in a blender and blend until smooth.

## PINEAPPLE CARROT JUICE

Handful of cracked ice
4 carrots, coarsely chopped
½ pineapple (top and skin removed)

Put carrots and pineapple in a juicer. Take the juice and ice and put it into a blender. Blend well and serve.

Juices/Smoothies/Milks

## TOMATO FIRE

2 C. tomato juice
¼ Tbs. of Nama Shoyu
1 small red chile, deseeded and chopped
1 scallion, trimmed and chopped
6 ice cubes, crushed

Place all ingredients in a blender and blend well. Serve and enjoy!

## MINT, LIME AND CUCUMBER FRESCA

Few sprigs of mint
½ C. lime juice
1 cucumber, thinly sliced
1 C. water
1 packet of electroyletes
Ice cubes

Place all ingredients in a blender and mix well. Serve chilled.

## GREEN TEA SMOOTHIE

2 ¼ C. water
1 C. ice
1 green tea bag
8 C. loose bok choy
1 C. celery
4 C. frozen mixed berries

Make 1 cup of green tea. Steep green tea bag in hot water for 5 minutes. Add tea and remaining ingredients to a blender and blend well. Serve immediately.

## BROCCOLI, CELERY AND KALE JUICE

2 stalks broccoli
½ kale leaf
½ celery stalk
1 lemon
½ inch ginger

Place all ingredients in a juicer. Pour over ice and serve.

## CABBAGE AND CARROT JUICE

8 cabbage leaves
6 carrots
½ inch ginger

Place all ingredients in a juicer and serve immediately.

## GREEN APPLE CUCUMBER

2 large cucumbers
1 lemon
1 apple

Place all ingredients in a juicer and serve immediately.

## BERRY GREEN SMOOTHIE

2 ¾ C. ice
2 heads green leaf lettuce
1 inch ginger
1 lemon, juiced
2 C. pineapple, frozen in chunks
2 C. frozen mixed berries

Place all ingredients in a blender and blend until smooth. Serve immediately.

## GREEN LIFE JUICE

1 green apple
½ bunch spinach
4 kale leaves
¼ inch ginger

Place all ingredients in a juicer and serve immediately.

## BEET IT JUICE

2 beets
1 large carrot or 2 medium carrots
½ green apple
½ cucumber
3 celery stalks
1 small piece of ginger
¼ bunch spinach

Place all ingredients in a juicer and serve immediately.

## GREEN STAR SMOOTHIE

3 cups water
½ bunch cilantro
2 inch ginger, peeled
spinach and/or collard
2 star fruit, coarsely chopped
1 lime juiced
2 pears or apples
2 cups frozen mixed berries

Place all ingredients in a blender and blend well. Serve immediately.

## BROCCOLI BLAST

6 carrots
3 celery stalks
1 broccoli stalk
1 cucumber

Place all ingredients in a juicer and serve immediately.

## NUT MILK 1

1 C. almonds, brazil nuts, macadamia nut, etc
1 tsp. sea salt
2 C. water

Place all ingredients in a blender. Strain through nut milk bag. Chill and serve. You can save the remaining pulp, dehydrate it and use it as flour for other recipes.

## NUT MILK 2

1 cup almonds, brazil nuts, macadamia nuts, etc
2 pitted dates
1 tsp. vanilla
1 Tbs. cinnamon
2 C. water

Place all ingredients in a blender. Strain through nut milk bag. Chill and serve. You can save the remaining pulp, dehydrate it and use it as flour for other recipes.

## MILK OF TAHINI

½ C. tahini
2 dates
3 C. water
⅛ tsp. sea salt

Place all ingredients in a blender and blend well. Serve immediately.

Juices/Smoothies/Milks

# DETOX SPECIAL

4 stalks celery
1 cucumber
½ bunch spinach
¼ ginger
1 lemon

Place all ingredients in a juicer and enjoy.

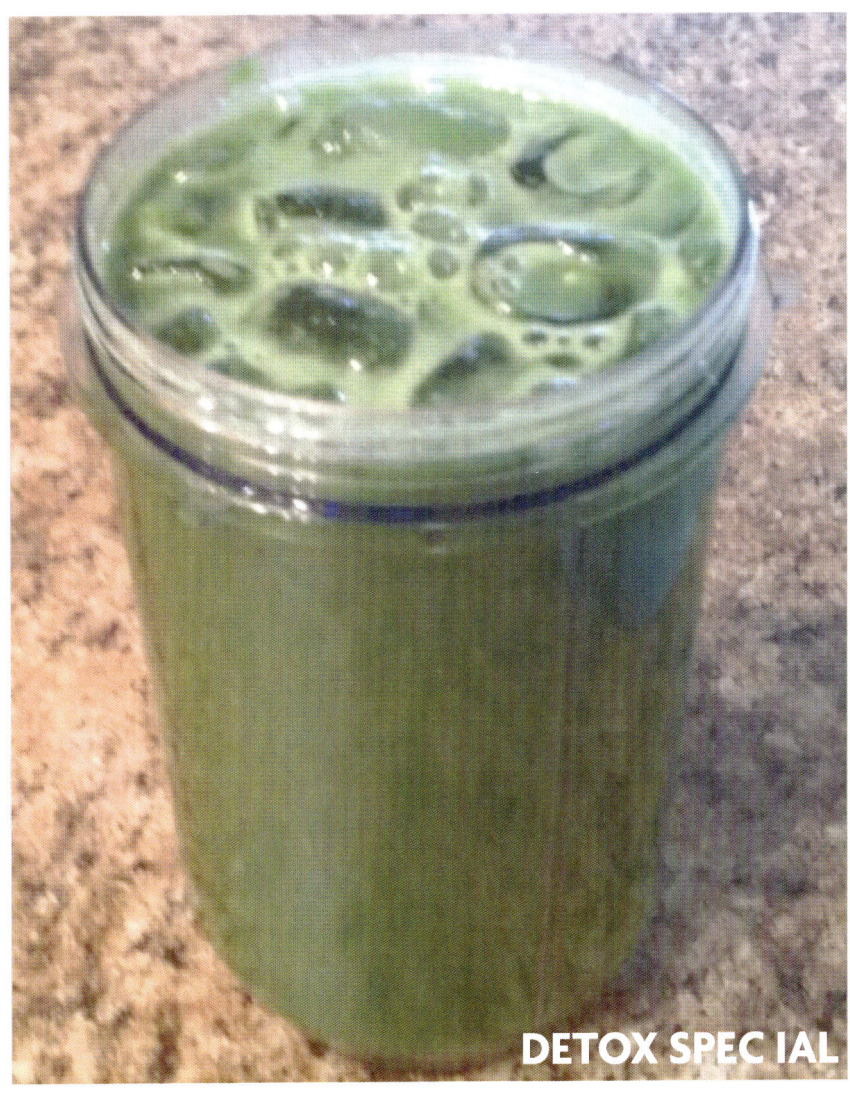

DETOX SPECIAL

## GREEN HEMP MILK

1 C. hemp seed
4 cups spinach
2 dates
1 Tbs. yacon syrup

Place all ingredients in a blender and blend well. Serve immediately. You can save the remaining pulp, dehydrate it and use it as flour for other recipes.

## MILK OF TAHINI

½ C. tahini
2 dates
3 C. water
⅛ tsp. sea salt

Place all ingredients in a blender and blend well. Serve immediately.

# Desserts

## FRENCH APPLE PIE

Crust:
2 C. almonds
⅓ C. yacon syrup
1 tsp. cinnamon
⅛ tsp. sea salt

For the Filling:
3 apples, peeled, cored and thinly sliced
2 Tbs. yacon syrup
1 tsp. cinnamon
⅛ tsp. nutmeg
1 lemon zested and juiced
¼ cup raisins

Put all ingredients for the crust in a food processor. Process well. Press mixture into a 9″ pie pan.

Put all the filling ingredients in a bowl and mix well. Spoon the mixture into the pie crust. Dehydrate 145° F for 3 hours or serve immediately.

## PISTACHIO HALVAH

1 C. raw tahini
¾ cup dates
¼ C. yacon syrup
¾ C. shelled pistachios, coarsely ground in a food processor

Place all ingredients in a bowl and mix thoroughly. Press the halvah into a glass dish. Coat with pistachios. Cover and store in the freezer. Serve thoroughly chilled, right out of the freezer.

## WALNUT FUDGE

3 C. walnuts
½ C. cacao powder
2 C. shredded coconut
2 tsp. vanilla
¾ C. yacon syrup
⅛ tsp. sea salt

Place walnuts in a food processor and chop finely. Place all ingredients in a bowl and mix well. Place the mixture in a glass dish, and layer about 1 inch thick. Cut into 1 inch squares. Place in freezer before serving or serve immediately.

## PUMPKIN PIE

Crust:
2 C. almonds
⅓ C. yacon syrup
1 tsp. cinnamon
⅛ tsp. sea salt

Put all ingredients for the crust in a food processor. Process well. Press mixture into a 9″ pie pan.

Filling:
2 C. cashews
1 C. coconut butter
2 C. carrot juice
¾ C. Yacon syrup
⅓ C. dates
1 Tbs. Vanilla
1 tsp. cinnamon
2 tsp. ginger
½ tsp. nutmeg
¾ tsp. sea salt

Place all filling ingredients in a food processor. Mix until smooth. Pour mixture into crust. Dehydrate at 145° for 3 hours and serve warm or put in freezer for 1 hour and serve.

# COCONUT-HAYSTACKS

½ C. cacao powder
3 C. shredded coconut
¾ C. coconut butter
½ C. yacon syrup
1 tsp. vanilla
⅛ tsp. sea salt

Place all ingredients in a bowl and mix well. In a medium mixing bowl, combine the carob powder and shredded coconut, and mix well. Add the coconut butter and agave nectar and mix well. Take a tablespoon of mixture and form into mounds. Freeze for at least 45 minutes before serving.

# PECAN PIE

Crust:
2 C. almonds
⅓ C. yacon syrup
1 tsp. cinnamon
⅛ tsp. sea salt

Place all ingredients for the crust in a food processor. Process well. Press mixture into a 9″ pie pan.

Filling:
⅓ cup coconut water
¼ cup pecans
½ cup raisins

Place all ingredients in a food processor and mix thoroughly. Spoon the mixture into the pie crust. Refrigerate or serve immediately.

# STRAWBERRY CREAM PIE

Crust:
2 C. almonds
⅓ C. yacon syrup
1 tsp. cinnamon
⅛ tsp. sea salt

For the Filling:
1 ½ cup strawberries
1 C cashew
¼ yacon syrup

Put all ingredients for the crust in a food processor. Process well. Press mixture into a 9″ pie pan.

Place all filling ingredients in a food processor. Mix until smooth. Pour mixture into crust. Top with chopped nuts. Dehydrate at 145° F for 3 hours and serve warm or refrigerate for 30 minutes or serve immediately.

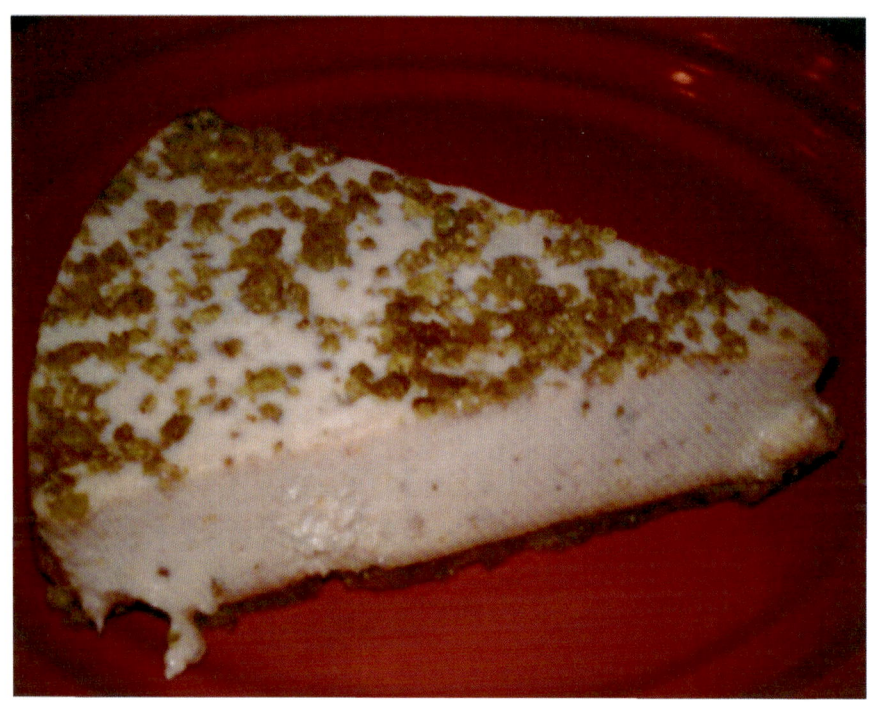

## ALMOND SMASH MACAROONS

2 C. dried coconut
¼ C. almonds, chopped
¼ C. almond pulp
½ C. dried cherries, chopped
½ C. yacon syrup
¼ C. coconut butter

Place all ingredients into a food processor and blend until it takes on the consistency of dough. Scoop out 1 tablespoon of the mixture and place on a mesh dehydrator sheet. Dehydrate at 115° F for 12 hours. Serve and enjoy!

## CINNAMON GINGER TRUFFLES

2 C. almonds, ground fine or almond pulp
1 Tbs. cinnamon
1 tsp. ginger
½ tsp. nutmeg
¼ tsp. cloves
½ C. yacon syrup
½ C. dried cranberries
½ C. raisins

Place almonds in coffee grinder or food processor until finely ground. Add spices and combine. Add cranberries and raisins and pulse for several seconds. Add remaining ingredients and blend well. Take 1 tablespoon of mixture and roll into balls. Roll into balls. Place in refrigerator for 20 minutes and serve.

## PERSIMMON PIE

Crust:
2 C. almonds
⅓ C. yacon syrup
1 tsp. cinnamon
⅛ tsp. sea salt

Filling:
2 persimmons
1 C. almond milk
⅛ tsp. sea salt
1 tsp. cinnamon

Put all ingredients for the crust in a food processor. Process well. Press mixture into a 9″ pie pan.

Place all filling ingredients in a food processor. Mix until smooth. Pour mixture into crust. Dehydrate at 145° F for 3 hours and serve warm or serve immediately.

## CINNAMON ALMOND RAISIN COOKIES

2 C. almonds, ground or almond pulp
1 apple, deseeded
½ C. coconut butter
¼ C. yacon syrup
1 Tbs. cinnamon
1 C. raisins

Place all ingredients in a food processor and mix until you achieve the consistency of dough. Scoop out 1 tablespoon of mixture and form into the shape of a cookie. Place cookie on mesh dehydrator sheet and dehydrate at 115° F for 8 hours.

# STRAWBERRY CHEESECAKE

Crust:
2 C. almonds
⅓ C. yacon syrup
1 tsp. cinnamon
⅛ tsp. sea salt

For the Filling:
2 C. soaked cashews
½ lemon juice
½ tsp. Salt
1 tsp. cinnamon
2 Tbs. vanilla
¼ C. yacon syrup
2 Tbs. coconut butter

Strawberry Sauce:
8 Strawberries
1 Tbs. coconut butter
1 tsp. cinnamon
1 tsp. vanilla
⅛ tsp. sea salt

Toppings:
4 strawberries, sliced

Put all ingredients for the crust in a food processor. Process well. Press mixture into a 9″ pie pan.

Place ingredients for filling in a food processor and mix well. Pour filling into a glass container and cover with cheese cloth for 4 hours. Pour into pie pan.

Place ingredients for strawberry sauce in a blender and blend well. Pour into pie pan with filling.

Shake pie around gently to mix sauce and filling.

Top with sliced strawberries. Freeze for 30 minutes and serve.

## ORANGE SORBET

2 C. orange, deseeded
½ C. yacon syrup
1 C. brazil nut milk (see recipe)
½ tsp. cinnamon
⅛ tsp. sea salt

Place all ingredients in blender and blend well until you achieve a smooth consistency. Pour mixture into an ice cream freezer and freeze according to ice cream maker's directions. Enjoy!

## CHOCOLATE MOUSSE

¾ C. dates soaked and pitted
2 avocados
1 C. almond milk (see Almond Milk recipe)
¾ C. cacao powder
½ C. yacon syrup

Place all ingredients into a food processor and mix well. Top with your favorite nuts. Refrigerate for 10 minutes or enjoy immediately.

# CHOCOLATE AVO-PUDDING

2 avocado
2 Tbs. coconut butter
4 Tbs. cacao powder
¼ C. yacon syrup
8 drops of stevia
1 tsp. vanilla powder or extract
1 tsp. cinnamon
⅛ tsp. sea salt

Place all ingredients in a food processor or blender and mix well. Chill for 10 minutes or serve immediately. Top with chopped almonds or fruit.

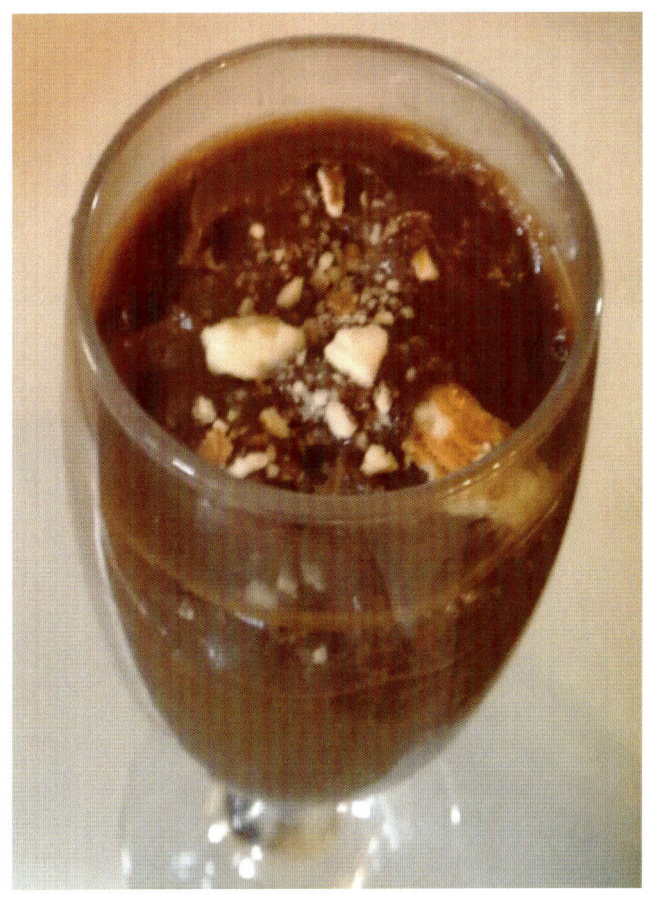

## APPLE CINNAMON GLAZE PIE

For the Crust:
2 C. almonds
⅓ C. yacon syrup
1 tsp. cinnamon
⅛ tsp. sea salt

Put all ingredients for the crust in a food processor. Process well. Press mixture into a 9″ pie pan.

For the Filling:
4 apples, peeled, cored and thinly sliced
½ lemon juiced
¼ C. Yacon syrup
1 tsp. cinnamon
⅓ C. almonds ground, or almond pulp

Place ingredients for filling in a food processor and blend gently where apple chunks are still present. Pour filling into crust and place in the dehydrator at 145° F for 3 hours.

## CINNAMON GLAZE

1 Tbs. coconut butter
3 Tbs. yacon syrup
½ tsp. cinnamon

Place all ingredients together in a bowl and mix thoroughly. Pour cinnamon glaze over pie filling. Reduce temperature to 115° F for an additional 4 hours.

# Soups

## HERBED TOMATO SOUP

1 medium tomato
1 large stalk celery
½ red pepper
¼ avocado
1 handful fresh basil
1 handful fresh parsley
1 Tbs. lemon juice
½ clove garlic
sea salt, to taste

Blend all ingredients until smooth, adding hot water for consistency. Adjust seasonings.

## CREAM OF CUCUMBER SOUP

4 Romaine lettuce leaves, chopped
1 cucumber, peeled, seeded, and chopped
1 C. warm water
1 Tbs. lemon juice
2 cloves garlic, minced
½ ripe avocado, chopped
2 Tbs. extra virgin olive oil

Place all ingredients in a blender and blend well. Serve and enjoy!

## THAI COCONUT SOUP

½ C. water
14 oz. coconut milk
1 zucchini, chopped (about 1 cup)
1 stalk celery, chopped
1 Tbs. lemon juice
1 tsp. mellow white miso
½ tsp. crushed garlic (1 clove)
¼ tsp. sea salt
dash cayenne pepper
1 Tbs. olive oil
½ avocado, chopped
1 Tbs. fresh minced dill, or 1 tsp. dried

Place all of the ingredients except the olive oil, avocado and dill in a blender. Blend until smooth.
Add the olive oil and avocado and blend until smooth. Add the dill and blend briefly just to mix.

## TOM KAI NO-GAI

14 oz. coconut milk
2 Tbs. of brown miso
14 oz. warm water
1 stalk fresh lemongrass, cut in 1-in pieces
1 C. sliced mushrooms (reishi, shiitake, maitake, portobello)
2 Tbs. fresh lime juice
¼ C. fresh basil leaves
6 qtr. slices of fresh ginger
¼ C. fresh cilantro
2 Tbs. thai chilli powder

Mix brown miso and 4 oz. of warm water together in a large bowl. Add other ingredients to same bowl and mix. Add 10 oz. of warm water at the end to create a warm soup and mix.

## CREME OF ZUCCHINI

½ cup water
1 zucchini, chopped (about 1 cup)
1 stalk celery, chopped
1 Tbs. lemon juice
1 Tbs. yellow white miso
½ tsp. crushed garlic (1 clove)
¼ tsp. sea salt
dash cayenne pepper
1 Tbs. olive oil
½ avocado, chopped
1 Tbs. fresh minced dill, or 1 tsp. dried

Place all of the ingredients except the olive oil, avocado and dill in a blender. Blend until smooth.
Add the olive oil and avocado and blend until smooth. Add the dill and blend briefly just to mix.

## ITALIAN SPINACH SOUP

2 C. spinach
1 stalk celery
1 tomato
⅓ C. parsley, chopped
¼ C. basil, chopped
¼ avocado
1 small clove garlic
1 tsp. lemon juice
1 tsp. apple cider vinegar
2 Tbs. extra virgin olive oil
¼ tsp. dry oregano
1 tsp. sea salt

Place all ingredients in a blender and blend well. Serve and enjoy!

# CREAM OF BROCCOLI SOUP

2 avocados
8 C. broccoli florets, chopped
¼ red onion, chopped
1 clove garlic
3 Tbs. Nama Shoyu or Bragg Liquid Aminos
⅛ tsp. sea salt
2 C. warm to hot water
2 Tbs. extra virgin olive oil
⅛ tsp. ground black pepper

Place ingredients in a blender. Add water and blend into a creamy soup.

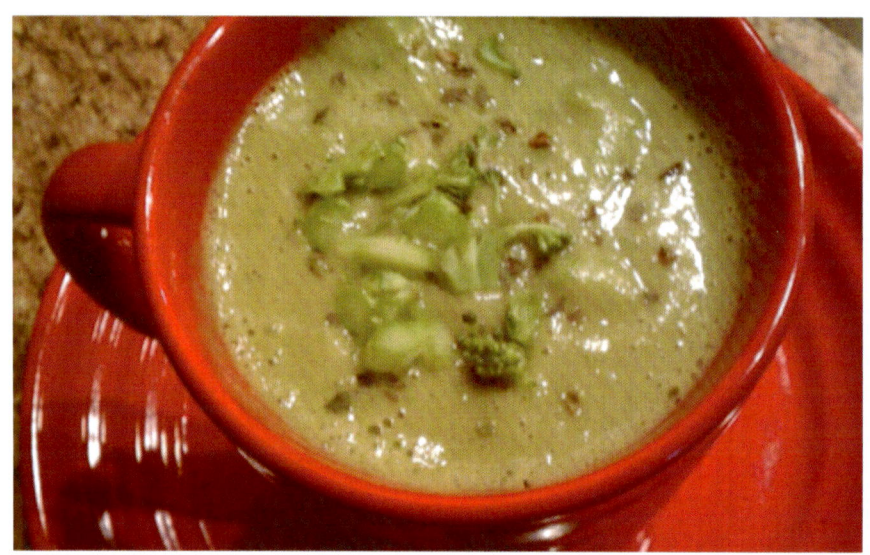

## CREAMY AVOCADO SOUP

1 cucumber, peeled
⅓ C. fresh cilantro, chopped
⅓ C. fresh parsley, chopped
2 cloves of garlic, minced
1 tsp. ginger powder
¼ C. Nama Shoyu or ¼ C. Bragg Liquid Aminos
⅓ C. extra virgin olive oil
1 C. lemon juice
4 avocados peeled and seeded
1 medium tomato
1 C. warm to hot water

Place all ingredients in a blender and blend. Serve and enjoy. Blend less for a hearty and chunky soup.

## CREAM OF SPINACH SOUP

2 C. spinach, chopped
1 avocado
1 C. warm to hot water
2 cloves garlic, minced
1 tsp. ginger powder
2 shallots, chopped
¼ C. Nama Shoyu, or ¼ C. Bragg Liquid Aminos
2 Tbs. lime juice
⅓ C. cilantro, chopped
½ C. extra virgin olive oil
½ C. portobello mushrooms, thinly sliced.

Place all ingredients except mushrooms in a blender and blend well. Garnish with mushrooms and serve.

## TOMATO BISQUE

- 4 medium tomatoes
- 2 Tbs. dark miso
- 1 Tbs. yacon syrup or 5 drops stevia
- 1 tsp. sea salt
- 1 bay leaf
- ¼ tsp. dried basil
- ¼ tsp. ground black pepper
- ¼ C. extra virgin olive oil
- ⅓ C. ground almonds

Place all ingredients in a blender and blend thoroughly. Dehydrate at 145° F for 3 hours. Serve warm.

# Breads/Crackers/Crust/Chips

## PIZZA CRUST (MAKES 2 CRUSTS)

2 C. ground sunflower seeds
1 C. ground flax seed
1 small tomato
¼ red onion
¼ C. extra virgin olive oil
½ C. water
½ tsp. salt
½ tsp. thyme

Place ingredients into a food processor and mix. Process until it forms dough. Add water to create a dough consistency. Remove dough and place on a Teflex sheet. Sprinkle water over dough and use the palm of hand to form the dough into shape of a pizza with outside edge of 1 ½ inch thickness. Place in dehydrator at 115° F for 6 hours. Slide crust off of Teflex onto mesh sheet and dehydrate at 115° F for another 6 hours. After done fill with pizza ingredients.

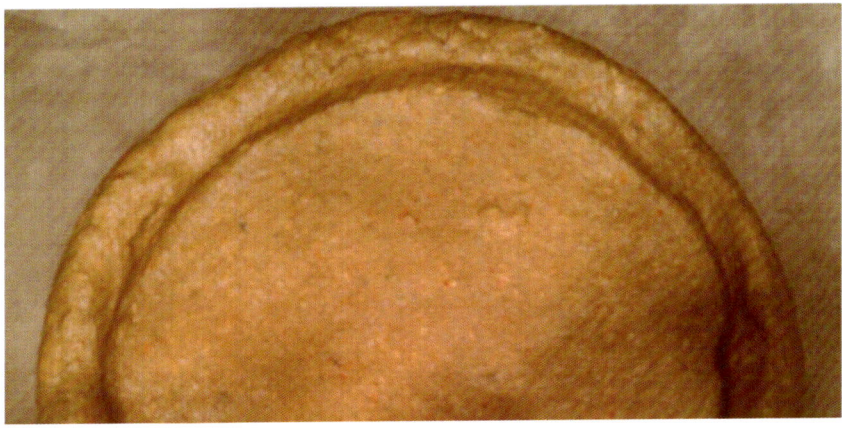

## ONION BREAD

3 yellow onions
1 ½ C. flax seed, ground
½ C. sunflower seed, ground
½ C. Nama Shoyu or Bragg Liquid Aminos
¼ C. extra virgin olive oil

Peel onions and slice thinly by hand or use slicing disc of food processor.

Grind sunflower seeds and flax seeds into a powder with a coffee grinder or food processor. Pour seed flour into a bowl and add the other ingredients.

Spoon out mixture onto Teflex sheet and spread it out with a ¼ inch thickness. Dehydrate at 115° F for 6 hours and then flip bread onto a mesh dehydrator tray and dehydrate at 115° F for an additional 6 hours. Slice into squares and use the bread for sandwiches.

## ALMOND CINNAMON RAISIN BREAD

6 C. almonds, ground or almond pulp
2 C. flax seed, ground
1 C. extra virgin olive oil
½ C. yacon syrup or 1 C. dates
1 Tbs. cinnamon
1 C. raisins
1 tsp. sea salt

Grind almonds and flax seeds into a powder with a coffee grinder or food processor. Pour flour into a bowl and add the other ingredients and mix well. Spoon out mixture onto Teflex sheet and spread it out to have a ¼ inch thickness. Dehydrate at 115° F for 6 hours and then flip bread onto a mesh dehydrator tray and dehydrate at 115° F for an additional 6 hours. Slice into squares and serve almond butter.

## FLAX CRACKERS

2 C. flax seeds
1 red bell pepper
¾ C. sun-dried tomatoes
1 fresh tomatoes
1 lemon juiced
1 clove garlic
½ onion, chopped

Place all ingredients in food processor and mix thoroughly. Place mixture on a Teflex sheet and spread it out to have a ¼ inch thickness. Dehydrate at 115° F for 6 hours and then flip crackers onto a mesh dehydrator tray and dehydrate at 115° F for an additional 6 hours.

## ZUCCHINI BREAD

2 C. flax seed, ground
1 C. pecans, ground
1 ½ C. raisins
1 C. zucchini
2 tsp. cinnamon
1 tsp. vanilla
½ tsp. nutmeg
1 tsp. sea salt

Grind almonds and flax seeds into a powder with a coffee grinder or food processor. Pour flour into a bowl and add the other ingredients and mix well. Spoon out mixture onto Teflex sheet and spread it out to have a ¼ inch thickness. Dehydrate at 115° F for 6 hours and then flip bread onto a mesh dehydrator tray and dehydrate at 115° F for an additional 6 hours. Slice into squares and serve almond butter.

## TORTILLAS

2 large carrots, chopped
2 zucchini (green or yellow), chopped
2 avocados, peeled and pitted
1 tsp. sea salt
1 Tbs. lemon juice
¼ onion, sliced
1 clove garlic
2 C. flax seed

Grind flax seeds into a powder with a coffee grinder or food processor. Put flax powder and remaining ingredients in a food processor and mix thoroughly. Spoon mixture onto Teflex sheet and spread it out to have a ¼ inch thickness. Dehydrate at 115° F for 3 hours. Slice into squares and serve. Use as shells for tacos or fajitas.

## VEGGIE CRACKERS

½ onion, chopped
2 cloves garlic
½ bunch spinach
1 C. cilantro
1 tomato
1 tsp. sea salt
⅓ C. lemon juice
2 zucchini, shredded
1 C. flax seed, whole
2 C. flax seed, ground

Place onion, garlic, spinach, tomato, herbs, sea salt and lemon juice in a blender and blend well. Pour the mixture into a bowl and add in the zucchini, flax seeds, and carrots. Mix ingredients together well. Spoon mixture onto Teflex sheet and spread it out to have a ¼ inch thickness. Dehydrate at 105° F for 12 hours.

## PIZZA CRACKERS

1 C. flax seed
2 Tbs. white miso
2 red bell peppers, stem and seeds removed
2 broccoli heads
2 stalks celery
2 medium tomatoes
½ red onion
½ tsp. sea salt

Grind flax seeds into a powder with a coffee grinder or food processor. Put flax powder and remaining ingredients in a food processor and mix thoroughly. Spoon mixture onto Teflex sheet and spread it out to have a ¼ inch thickness. Dehydrate at 115° F for 6 hours and then flip crackers onto a mesh dehydrator tray and dehydrate at 115° F for an additional 6 hours.

# CHEESY KALE CHIPS

1 head of kale, remove leaves from stem
2 Tbs. extra virgin olive oil
½ red bell pepper
½ C. cashews, soaked
1 lemon, juiced
¼ C. water

Place all ingredients except for kale in a blender and blend well. Place kale leaves in a bowl and pour blended mixture over it. Toss and mix well. Place mixture on mesh dehydrator sheet and dehydrate at 105° F for 12 hours.

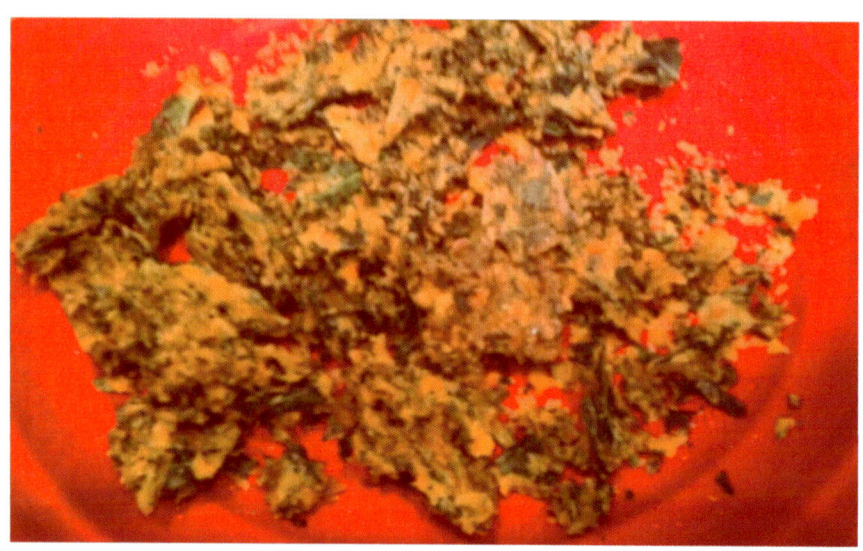

# THE GOOD CRACKER

- 1 C. sunflower seeds, ground
- 1 C. almonds, ground or almond pulp
- 1 tomato
- ½ red onion, sliced
- 3 Tbs. flax seed
- 3 tsp. cumin seed
- 1 tsp. sea salt

Grind sunflower seeds, flax seeds, and almonds into flour with a coffee grinder or food processor. Put flax, sunflower and almond flour and remaining ingredients in a food processor and mix thoroughly. Spoon mixture onto Teflex sheet and spread it out to have a ¼ inch thickness. Dehydrate at 115° F for 6 hours and then flip crackers onto a mesh dehydrator tray and dehydrate at 115° F for an additional 12 hours.

# KALE CHIPS

- 1 head of kale, remove leaves from stem
- 2 Tbs. extra virgin olive oil
- ⅛ tsp. sea salt

Place kale in a bowl and add olive oil and salt. Mix thoroughly. Place mixture on mesh dehydrator sheet and dehydrate at 105° F for 12 hours.

## SALT AND VINEGAR FLAX CRACKERS

2 cups flax seeds
½ C. apple cider vinegar
1 lemon, juiced
1 Tbsp garlic powder
2 tsp. sea salt

Soak flax seeds in vinegar, lemon juice, and garlic powder for 30 minutes or more. Spoon mixture onto Teflex sheet and spread it out to have a ¼ inch thickness. Sprinkle crackers with sea salt and dehydrate at 115° F for 6 hours and then flip crackers onto a mesh dehydrator tray and dehydrate at 115° F for an additional 12 hours.

## SPICY FLAX CRACKERS

3 C. flax seeds, soaked at least 4 hours
1 Tbs. mustard seeds
1 green onion, chopped
1 clove garlic, chopped
2 Tbs. Nama Shoyu or Bragg Liquid Aminos

Grind mustard seeds in a coffee grinder. Put flax and remaining ingredients in a food processor and mix thoroughly. Spoon mixture onto Teflex sheet and spread it out to have a ¼ inch thickness. Dehydrate at 115° F for 6 hours and then flip crackers onto a mesh dehydrator tray and dehydrate at 115° F for an additional 12 hours.

# SUN-DRIED TOMATO CRACKERS

2 cups walnuts, soaked
4 zucchini, diced
½ C. sun-dried tomatoes, soaked
½ red bell pepper, chopped
1 C. flax seed, ground
⅓ C. lemon juice
1 tsp. sea salt
½ C. water

Grind walnuts and flax seeds into flour with a coffee grinder or food processor. Put walnut, flax flour, and remaining ingredients in a food processor and mix thoroughly. Add water slowly to achieve a dough consistency. Spoon mixture onto Teflex sheet and spread it out to have a ¼ inch thickness. Dehydrate at 115° F for 6 hours and then flip crackers onto a mesh dehydrator tray and dehydrate at 115° F for an additional 12 hours.

## SUN-DRIED TOMATO OLIVE CRACKERS

2 C. walnuts, soaked
½ C. ground flax
½ C. water
⅓ C. sun-dried tomatoes, soaked
½ C. olives, sliced
⅛ tsp. sea salt

Grind walnuts and flax seed into flour with a coffee grinder or food processor. Put flax, walnuts, and remaining ingredients in a food processor and mix thoroughly. Spoon mixture onto Teflex sheet and spread it out to have a ¼ inch thickness. Dehydrate at 115° F for 6 hours and then flip crackers onto a mesh dehydrator tray and dehydrate at 115° F for an additional 12 hours.

## ONION FLAX CRACKERS

2 C. flax seeds soaked at least 4 hours
1 C. ground flax seeds
1 yellow onion, chopped
1 clove garlic, chopped
¼ C. Nama Shoyu

Grind 1 C. of flax with a coffee grinder. Put ground flax seed, soaked flax seed, and remaining ingredients in a food processor and mix thoroughly. Spoon mixture onto Teflex sheet and spread it out to ¼ inch thickness. Dehydrate at 115° F for 6 hours and then flip crackers onto a mesh dehydrator tray and dehydrate at 115° F for an additional 12 hours.

# BIBLIOGRAPHY

*A Brief History of Raw Milk.* January 7, 2012. www.raw-milk-facts.com.

Agur, Anne M.R., and Arthur F. Dalley II. *Grants Atlas of Anatomy.* 11. Baltimore, Maryland: Lippincott Williams and Wilkins, 2005.

Aiello, LP, J Wong, J Cavallerano, SE Bursell, and LM Aiello. "Retinopathy." In *Handbook of Exercise in Diabetes*, by N Ruderman, JT Devlin and A Kriska, 401-413. Alexandria, VA: American Diabetes Association, 2002.

Akerfeldt, Mia C., and Ross D. Laybutt. "Inhibition of Id1 Augments Insulin Secretion and Protects Against High-Fat Diet-Induced Glucose Intolerance." *Diabetes* 60, no. 10 (October 2011): 2506-2514.

Althuis, MD, NE Jordan, EA Ludington, et al. "Glucose and insulin responses to dietary chromium supplements: a meta-analysis." *American Journal of Clinical Nutrition* 76, no. 1 (2002): 148-155.

American Diabetes Association. "Diagnosis and Classification of Diabetes Mellitus." *Diabetes Care* 33, no. Suppl. 1 (2010): S62-S69.

American Diabetes Association. *Intensive Diabetes Management.* Alexandria, Virginia.

American Diabetes Association. *Medical Management of Type 1 Diabetes.* Alexandria, Virginia.

American Diabetes Association. *Medical Management of Type 2 Diabetes.* Alexandria, Virginia.

American Foundation. *American Medicine.* Vol. II. New York, New York: The American Foundation, 1937.

Anderson, Odin W. *State Enabling Legislation for Non-Profit Hospital and Medical Plans.* Ann Arbor: University of Michigan Press, 1944.

Anderson, RJ, et al. "Anxiety and poor glycemic control: a meta-analytic review of the literature." *Int J Psychiatry Med* 32 (2002): 235-247.

Appel, LJ, et al. "A clinical trial of the effects of dietary patterns on blood pressure. DASH Collaborative Research Group." *New England Journal of Medicine* 336 (1997): 1117-1124.

Balk, EM, A Tatsioni, AH Lichtenstein, et al. "Effect of chromium supplementation on glucose metabolism and lipids: A systematic review of randomized controlled trials." *Diabetes Care* 30, no. 8 (2007): 2154-2163.

Barbour, M.G., J.H. Burk, and W.D. Pitts. *Terrestrial Plant Ecology*. Menlo Park, California: The Benjamin/Cummings Publishing Company, 1980.

Barnard, ND, et al. "A low-fat vegan diet improves glycemic control and cardiovascular risk factors in a randomized clinical trial in individuals with Type 2 Diabetes." *Diabetes Care* 29 (2006): 1777-1783.

Bax, JJ, LH Young, RL Frye, RO Bonow, HO Steinberg, and EJADA Barrett. "Screening for coronary artery disease in patients with diabetes." *Diabetes Care* 30 (2007): 2729-2736.

Berger, M, et al. "Metabolic and hormonal effects of muscular exercise in juvenile type diabetes." *Diabetologica* 13 (1977): 355-365.

"Beyond Vegetarianism." http://www.beyondveg.com/nicholson-w/hb/hb-interview1c.shtml.

Bonadkdar, RA, and E Guarneri. "Coenzyme Q10." *American Family Physician* 72, no. 6 (2005): 1065-1069.

Boule, NG, E Haddad, GP Kenny, GA Wells, and RJ Sigal. "Effects of exercise on glycemic control and body mass in Type 2 Diabetes mellitus: a meta-analysis of controlled clinical trials." *Journal of the American Medical Association* 286 (2001): 1218-1227.

# Bibliography

Boule, NG, GP Kenny, E Haddad, GA Wells, and RJ Sigal. "Meta-analysis of the effect of structured exercise training on cardiorespiratory fitness in Type 2 Diabetes mellitus." *Diabetologia* 46 (2003): 1071-1081.

Campbell, Amy P. "Diabetes and Dietary Supplements." *Clinical Diabetes* 28, no. 1 (January 2010): 35-39.

Campbell, T. Colin, and Thomas M. Campbell. *The China Study: The Most Comprehensive Study of Nutrition Ever Conducted and the Startling Implications for Diet, Weight Loss and Long-term Health.* Kent Town: Wakefield Press, 2007.

Canner, PL, et al. "Fifteen year mortality in Coronary Drug Project patients: long-term benefit with niacin." *J Am Coll Cardiol* 8 (1986): 1245-1255.

Castaneda, C, et al. "A randomized controlled trial of resistance exercise training to improve glycemic control in older adults with Type 2 Diabetes." *Diabetes Care* 25 (2002): 2335-2341.

Cauza, E, et al. "The relative benefits of endurance and strength training on the metabolic factors and muscle function of people with Type 2 Diabetes mellitus." *Arch Phys Med Rehabil* 86 (2005): 1527-1533.

Centers for Medicaid and Medicare Services. Statistics. February 15, 2012. http://ems.gov/statistics.

"Chromium." *Office of Dietary Supplements.* www.ods.od.nih.gov/factsheets/chromium.asp (accessed April 14, 2012).

Colberg, SR, et al. "Exercise and Type 2 Diabetes: the American College of Sports Medicine and the American Diabetes Association: joint position statement." *Diabetes Care* 33 (2010): 2692-2696.

*Complete Blood Count.* http://labtestsonline.org/understanding/analytes/cbc/tab/test (accessed September 6, 2011).

**The Raw Truth: The Recipe for Reversing Diabetes**

*Comprehensive Metabolic Panel.* April 29, 2011. http://labtestsonline.org/understanding/analytes/emp/.

*Concerned about Enzymes and the Excalibur Thermostat Control.* March 28, 2012. http://www.excaliburdehydrator.com.

Cousens, Gabriel. *Rainbow Green Live-Food Cuisine.* Berkeley: North Atlantic Books, 2003.

Cowie, CC, et al. "Prevalence of diabetes and high risk for diabetes using A1C. criteria in the U.S. population in 1988-2006." *Diabetes Care* 33 (2010): 562-568.

Dalrymple, G. Brent. "The age of the Earth in the twentieth century: a problem (mostly) solved." *Special Publications, Geological Society of London* 190, no. 1: 205-221.

Daniel, CR, AJ Cross, C. Koebnick, and R Sinha. "Trends in meat consumption in the USA." *Public Health and Nutrition* 14, no. 4 (April 2011): 575-83.

Deacon, HJ. "Guide to Klaises River." http://academic.sun.ac.za/archaeology/KRguide2001.pdf (accessed March 4, 2007).

DeFronzo, Ralph A. "From the Triumvirate to the Ominous Octet: A New Paradigm for the Treatment of Type 2 Diabetes Mellitus." *Diabetes* 58, no. 4 (April 2009): 773-795.

Delahanty, LM, et al. "Association of diabetes-related emotional distress with diabetes treatment in primary care patients with Type 2 Diabetes." *Diabetic Medicine* 24 (2007): 48-54.

Dodson, Aidan. *Monarchs of the Nile.* Rubicon Press, 1995.

Dunstan, DW, et al. "High-intensity resistance training improves glycemic control in older patients with Type 2 Diabetes." *Diabetes Care* 25 (2002): 1729-1736.

# Bibliography

*Early Man 'Couldn't Stomach Milk'.* January 5, 2012. http://news.bbc.co.uk/2/hi/health/6397001.stm.

Economic Research Service (ERS), U.S. Department of Agriculture (USDA). *Food Availability (Per Capita) Data System.* http://www.ers.usda.gov/Data/FoodConsumption.

Eilers, Robert D. *Regulation of Blue Cross and Blue Shield Plans.* Homewood, Illinois: Richard D. Irwin, Inc., 1963.

Expert Committee on the Diagnosis and Classification of Diabetes Mellitus. "Report of the Expert Committee on the Diagnosis and Classification of Diabetes Mellitus." *Diabetes Care* 20 (1997): 1183-1197.

Faulkner, Edwin J. *Health Insurance.* New York, New York: McGraw-Hill, 1960.

*Fenugreek (Trigonella foenum-graecum L. Leguminosae).* February 22, 2012. www.naturalstandard.com.

*Fenugreek.* February 22, 2012. www.naturaldatabase.com.

Foster, GD, et al. "A randomized trial of a low-carbohydrate diet for obesity." *New England Journal of Medicine* 348 (2003): 2082-2090.

Foster, GD, et al. "Weight and metabolic outcomes after 2 years on a low-carbohydrate versus low-fat diet: a randomized trial." *Annals of Internal Medicine* 153 (2010): 147-157.

Franz, MJ, et al. "Evidence-based nutrition principles and recommendations for the treatment and prevention of diabetes and related complications." *Diabetes Care* 25 (2002): 148-198.

Franz, MJ, et al. "Weight-loss outcomes: a systematic review and meta-analysis of weight-loss clinical trials with a minimum 1-year follow-up." *Journal of the American Dietary Association* 107 (2007): 1755-1767.

Gardner, CD, et al. "Comparison of the Atkins, Zone, Ornish, and LEARN diets for a change in weight and related risk factors among overweight premenopausal women: the A TO Z Weight Loss Study: a randomized trial." *Journal of the American Medical Association* 297 (2007): 969-977.

Grimal, Nicholas. *History of Ancient Egypt.* Blackwell, 1988.

Grossman, Charles J. *Blond's Medical Guides: Physiology.* New York, New York: Sulzburger & Graham Publishing, Ltd., 1995.

Group, Australian Carbohydrate Intolerance Study in Pregnant Women (ACHOIS) Trial. "Effect of gestational diabetes mellitus on pregnancy outcomes." *New England Journal of Medicine* 352 (2005): 2477-2486.

Group, Dietary Intervention Randomized Controlled Trial (DIRECT). "Weight loss with a low-carbohydrate, Mediterranean, or low-fat diet." *New England Journal of Medicine* 359 (2008): 229-241.

Group, Environmental Working. *Body burden: The pollution in people.* April 7, 2011. http://www.ewg.org/sites/bodyburden1/index.php.

Harper, Douglas. *Online Etymology Dictionary: diabetes.* (accessed 06 10, 2011).

Herman, SL, et al. "Four-week dynamic stretching warm-up intervention elicits longer-term performance benefits." *Journal of Strength and Conditioning Research* 4 (2008): 1286.

Huang, H-Y, B Caballero, S Chang, AJ Alberg, RD Semba, and C. Schneyer. *Evidence Report/Technology Assessment No. 139.* Evidence-based Practice Center, Johns Hopkins University, Agency for Healthcare Research and Quality, 2006.

*Important Dates in Milk History.* January 7, 2003. www.idfa.org.

*Institute of Medicine: Dietary Reference Intakes: Energy, Carbohydrate, Fiber, Fat, Fatty Acids, Cholesterol, Protein, and Amino Acids.* Washington, D.C.: National Academics Press.

International Expert Committee. "International Expert Committee report on the role of the AIC assay in the diagnosis of diabetes." *Diabetes Care*, 2009: 1327-1334.

Jouanna, J. *Hippocrates*. Baltimore, Maryland: Johns Hopkins University Press, 1999.

Katon, W, MY Fan, J Unutzer, J Taylor, H Pincus, and M Schoenbaum. "Depression and diabetes: a potentially lethal combination." *J Gen Intern Med* 23 (2008): 1571-1575.

Kim, J, G Formoso, and Y Li. "Epigallocatechin gallate, a green tea polyphenol, mediates NO-dependent vasodilation using signaling pathways in vascular endothelium requiring reactive oxygen species and Fyn." *Journal of Biological Chemistry* 282, no. 18 (2007): 13736-13747.

Klein, S, et al. "Weight management through lifestyle modification for the preention and management of Type 2 Diabetes: rationale and strategies: a statement of the American Diabetes Association, the North American Association for the Study of Obesity, and the American Society for Clinical Nutrition." *Diabetes Care* 27 (2004): 2067-2073.

Larsson, SC, and A Wolk. "Magnesium intake and risk of type 2 diabetes: a meta analysis." *Journal of Internal Medicine* 262, no. 2 (2007): 208-214.

Lemaster, JW, GE Reiber, DG Smith, PJ Heagerty, and C. Wallace. "Daily weight-bearing activity does not increase the risk of diabetic foot ulcers." *Med Sci Sports Exerc* 35 (2003): 1093-1099.

*Louis Pasteur (1822-1895)*. January 7, 2012. www.bbc.co.uk.

"Magnesium." *Office of Dietary Supplements Web site*. April 14, 2012. www.ods.od.nih.gov/factsheets/magnesium.asp.

Manhesa, Gerard, Claude Allegre, Bernard Duprea, and Bruno Hamelin. "Lead isotope study of basic ultrabasic layered complexes:

Speculations about the age of the earth and primitive mantle characteristics." *Earth and Planetary Science Letters* (Elsevier B.V.) 47, no. 3 (1980): 370-382.

Manning, RM, RT Jung, GP Leese, and RW Newton. "The comparison of four weight reduction strategies aimed at overweight patients with diabetes mellitus: four-year follow-up." *Diabetic Medicine* 15 (1998): 497-502.

McCrone, J. "Fired Up: Theory on when prehistoric man first used fire." *New Scientist*, May 2000.

McHugh, MP, et al. "To stretch or not to stretch: The role of stretching in injury prevention and performance." *Scandinavian Journal of Medicine and Science in Sports* 20 (2010): 169.

Metzger, BE, et al. "Hyperglycemia and adverse pregnancy outcomes." *New England Journal of Medicine* 358 (2008): 1991-2002.

Mogensen, CE. "Nephropathy." By Handbook of Exercise in Diabetes, edited by N Ruderman, JT Devlin and A Kriska. Alexandria, Virginia: American Diabetes Association, 2002.

Moore, Keith L, and Arthur F. Dalley. *Clinically Oriented Anatomy*. Fifth. Baltimore, Maryland: Lippincott Williams and Wilkins, 2006.

Network, Kennedy Shriver National Institute of Child Health and Human Development Maternal-Fetal Medicine Units. "A multicenter, randomized trial of treatment for mild gestational diabetes." *New England Journal of Medicine* 361 (2009): 1339-1348.

Nordmann, AJ, et al. "Effects of low-carbohydrate vs. low-fat diets on weight loss and cardiovascular risk factors: a meta-analysis of randomized controlled trials." *Arch Intern Med* 166 (2006): 285-293.

Norris, SL, et al. "Efficacy of pharmacotherapy for weight loss in adults with Type 2 Diabetes mellitus: a meta-analysis." *Arch Intern Med* 164 (2004): 1395-1404.

# Bibliography

Norris, SL, et al. "Long-term effectiveness of weight-loss interventions in adults with prediabetes: a review." *American Journal of Preventive Medicine* 28, no. 126-139 (2005).

O'Kane, MJ, B Bunting, M Copeland, and VE Coates. "Efficacy of self monitoring of blood glucose in patients with newly diagnosed Type 2 Diabetes (ESMON study): Randomised controlled trial." *BMJ* 336 (2008): 1174-1177.

Panel, International Association of Diabetes and Pregnancy Study Groups Consensus. "International association of diabetes and pregnancy study groups recommendations on the diagnosis and classification of hyperglycemia and pregnancy." *Diabetes Care* 33 (2010): 676-682.

Park, M.A. *Biological Anthropology.* Mountain View, California: Mayfield Publishing Company, 1999.

Peterson, DM, et al. *Overview of the benefits and risks of exercise.* February 4, 2012. http://www.uptodate.com/home/index.html.

Pi-Sunyer, X, et al. "Reduction in weight and cardiovascular disease risk factors in individuals with Type 2 Diabetes: one-year results of the look AHEAD trial." *Diabetes Care* 30 (2007): 1374-1383.

*Program History & Data.* January 9, 2012. www.schoolnutrition.org.

Pyne, Stephen J. *Fire: A Brief History.* 2001: University of Washington Press.

Rancour, J, et al. "The effects of intermittent stretching following a 4-week static stretching protocol: A randomized trial." *Journal of Strength and Conditioning Research* 8 (2009): 2217.

Reed, Louis S. *Blue Cross and Medical Service Plans.* Washington, D.C.: U.S. Public Health Service, 1947.

Rock, CL. "Multivitamin-multimineral supplements: who uses them?" *American Journal of Clinical Nutrition* 85 (2007): 277S-279S.

Rolland, Nicolas. "Was the Emergence of Home Bases and Domestic Fire a Punctuated Event? A Review of the Middle Pleistocene Record in Eurasia." *Asian Perspectives: the Journal of Archaeology for Asia and the Pacific* 248-280.

Rubins, HB, et al. "Gemfibrozil for the secondary prevention of coronary heart disease in men with low levels of high-density lipoprotein cholesterol. Veterans Affairs High-Density Lipoprotein Cholesterol Intervention Trial Study Group." *New England Journal of Medicine* 341 (1999): 410-418.

Salas-Salvado, J, et al. "Reduction in the Incidence of Type 2 Diabetes with the Mediterranean Diet: Results of the PREDIMED-Reus Nutrition Intervention Randomized Trial." *Diabetes Care* 34 (2010): 14-19.

Selvin, E, et al. "Glycated hemoglobin, diabetes, and cardiovascular risk in nondiabetic adults." *New England Journal of Medicine* 362 (2010): 800-811.

Shaw, Ian. *Oxford History of Ancient Egypt*. Oxford University Press, 2000.

Shaw, Ian, and Paul Nicholson. *The Dictionary of Ancient Egypt*. Harry N. Abrams, Inc., Publishers, 1995.

Shaw, Steve. *Maximize Your Gym Time: A Look at the Most Productive Muscle Building Exercises*. http://www.muscleandstrength.com/articles/maximize-gym-time-most-productive-muscle-building-exercises.html (accessed February 18, 2012).

Sigal, RJ, GP Kenny, DH Wasserman, and C. Castaneda-Sceppa. "Physical activity/exercise and Type 2 Diabetes." *Diabetes Care* 27 (2004): 2518-2539.

Singh, IM, MH Shishehbor, and BJ Ansell. "High-density lipoprotein as a therapeutic target: a systematic review." *Journal of the American Medical Association* 298 (2007): 786-798.

# Bibliography

*Smallpox a Great and Terrible Scourge.* January 5, 2012. http://www.nlm.nih.gov/exhibition/smallpox/.

Stern, L, et al. "The effects of low-carbohydrate versus conventional weight loss diets in severely obese adults: one-year follow-up of a randomized trial." *Annals of Internal Medicine* 140 (2004): 778-785.

Stewart, Alex. *5 Workouts for Every Body Part - A Beginner's Guide.* September 23, 2009. http://www.bodybuilding.com/fun/stewart-beginner-training-guide-main.htm (accessed March 1, 2012).

—. *Gaining muscle after 40: A Complete Beginner's Guide.* June 11, 2009. http://www.bodybuilding.com/fun/over_40_beginner_training.htm (accessed March 3, 2012).

Takeuchi, Y, T Miyamoto, T Kakizawa, S Shigematsu, and K Hashizume. "Insulin Autoimmune Syndrome possibly caused by alpha lipoic acid." *Internal Medicine* 46, no. 5 (2007): 237-239.

*The Discovery of Insulin.* April 14, 2012. http://www.nobelprize.org/educational/medicine/insulin/discovery-insulin.html.

*The National School Lunch Program Background and Development.* January 9, 2012. www.usda.gov.

Turner-McGrievy, GM, ND Barnard, J Cohen, DJ Jenkins, L Gloede, and AA Green. "Changes in nutrient intake and dietary quality among participants with Type 2 Diabetes following a low-fat vegan diet or a conventional diabetes diet for 22 weeks." *Journal of the American Dietary Association* 108 (2008): 1636-1645.

"U.S. Department of Health and Human Services: 2008 Physical Activity Guidelines for Americans." 2008. http://www.health.gov/paguidelines/guidelines/default.aspx (accessed December 2010).

U.S. Geological Survey. 1997. http://pubs.usgs.gov/gip/geotime/age.html (accessed 01 10, 2006).

University, Rice. *Antioxidants and free radicals*. 1996. http://www.rice.edu/~jenky/sports/antiox.html (accessed January 26, 2012).

Van Horn, L, et al. "The evidence for dietary prevention and treatment of cardiovascular disease." *Journal of the American Dietary Association* 108 (2008): 237-331.

Vinik, A, and T Erbas. "Neuropathy." In *Handbook of Exercise in Diabetes*, by N Ruderman, JT Devlin and A Kriska, 463-496. Alexandria, Virginia: American Diabetes Association, 2002.

Wackers, FJ, et al. "Detection of Ischemia in Asymptomatic Diabetics Investigators. Detection of silent myocardial ischemia in asymptomatic diabetic subjects: the DIAD study." *Diabetes Care* 27 (2004): 1954-1961.

Wiener, RS, DC Wiener, and RJ Larson. "Benefits and risks of tight glucose control in critically ill adults: a meta-analysis." *Journal of the American Medical Association* 300 (2008): 933-944.

Wing, RR, and Look AHEAD Research Group. "Long-term effects of a lifestyle intervention on weight and cardiovascular risk factors in individuals with Type 2 Diabetes mellitus: four-year results of the Look AHEAD trial." *Arch Intern Med* 170 (2010): 1566-1575.

Wolf, AM, et al. "Translating lifestyle intervention to practice in obese patients with Type 2 Diabetes: Improving Control with Activity and Nutrition (ICAN) study." *Diabetes Care* 27 (2004): 1570-1576.

World Cancer Research Fund/American Institute for Cancer Research. *Food, Nutrition, Physical Activity, and the Prevention of Cancer: a Global Perspective*. Washington, D.C.: American Institute for Cancer Research, 2007.

# Bibliography

Zhang, X, SL Norris, EW Gregg, YJ Cheng, G Beckles, and HS Kahn. "Depressive symptoms and mortality among persons with and without diabetes." *American Journal of Epidemiology* 161 (2005): 652-660.

Ziegler, D, et al. "Oral treatment with alpha-lipoic acid improves symptomatic diabetic polyneuropathy: the SYDNEY 2 trial." *Diabetes Care* 19, no. 11 (2006): 2635-2370.

Ziemer, DC, et al. "Glucose-independent, black-white differences in hemoglobin A1C. levels: a cross-sectional analysis of 2 studies." *Annals of Internal Medicine* 152 (2010): 770-777.